QUICK GUIDES
Baby & Toddler Food

B⊞XTREE

ADVICE TO THE READER
*Before following any dietary or nutritional advice contained in this book
it is recommended that you consult a doctor if your child suffers from
any health problems or special conditions or if you are in any doubt*

First published in Great Britain in 1994 by Boxtree Limited,
Broadwall House, 21 Broadwall, London SE1 9PL

Copyright © Liz Earle 1994
All rights reserved

The right of Liz Earle to be identified as Author of this Work has
been asserted by her in accordance with the Copyright, Designs and
Patents Act 1988

10 9 8 7 6 5 4 3 2 1

ISBN: 1 85283 544 3

Text design by Blackjacks
Cover design by Hammond Hammond

Except in the United States of America this book is sold subject to the
condition that it shall not, by way of trade or otherwise, be lent,
resold, hired out or otherwise circulated without the publisher's prior
consent in any form of binding or cover than that in which it is
published and without a similar condition including this condition
being imposed upon a subsequent purchaser

Printed and Bound in Great Britain by Cox & Wyman Ltd.,
Reading, Berkshire

A CIP catalogue entry for this book is available from
the British Library

Contents

Introduction and Acknowledgements	4
1. Food for Life	5
2. A Child's Nutrition	9
3. What to Give When	23
4. Recipes	45
5. Special Diets	86
6. Commercial Foods	91
Useful Addresses	109
Index	111

Introduction

I have written this guide as a mother of both a baby and toddler. We all care deeply for our children and want the very best for them. Unfortunately, when it comes to modern baby foods our children are frequently short-changed. It is so vital that our children receive the best possible nutrition in their early, formative years. With the help of this *Quick Guide* you will find out just how easy it is to feed your small ones with the right foods to build their healthy future. Many complex books have been written about weaning, childhood nutrition and welfare. This small book will guide you through the maze of information you need in a simple and straightforward way. I wish you and your family the very best of health both now – and for the years to come.

Liz Earle

ACKNOWLEDGEMENTS

I am grateful to Sarah Mobsby and Laura Hill, Norland NNEB for helping to produce this book. Also for the invaluable information from paediatrician Dr Stanley Rom, the Health Education Authority and The Food Commission. Grateful thanks are most certainly due to Grannie Annie for valuable recipe testing and my own Lily and Guy for their enthusiastic recipe tasting. I am also indebted to the talented team at Boxtree, Rosemary Sandberg, and Claire Bowles, Publicity, for their unfailing enthusiasm and support.

1
Food for Life

From the day a baby is born, our children need food to grow and develop. Their food not only enables a baby to live, but also determines the quality of life. Whatever you feed your baby contributes greatly to his or her health both now and in the future – and is a wonderful gift to be enjoyed.

Setting the Pattern

From day one you are setting the tastes and eating habits of another person. While your children are unable to took after themselves and make their own decisions, you decide these things instead. Is this really relevant, you might ask? The simple answer is yes! Give your baby a sweet tooth now and your child may always crave unhealthy sugary foods. According to the Health Education Council, 'A number of researchers provide evidence that children's early experience with food and learned behaviour in the family are crucial in the development of dietary patterns. Those dietary behaviour patterns developed in early childhood may persist into adolescence and adulthood.' But it is not just a danger of creating bad eating habits for adulthood which should affect what you decide to feed your baby; the food your baby eats *now* has a dramatic impact on health both present and future. The message is clear – it is never too early to start.

Diet and Health

So-called 'diseases of affluence' affect people in developed Western societies and are linked to poor nutrition. These include heart disease and high blood pressure, diet-related cancers, obesity, late-onset diabetes and also an increased risk of strokes. The NHS spends more than £1 billion every year coping with the effects of our poor diet. Over 35 million working days are lost every year for diet-related sickness, not counting days taken and not certified, plus all those millions of half-days taken for visits to the dentist. This figure includes only directly related illnesses and does not take into account such factors as a poor diet increasing our risk to infections. There are also countless people who suffer from minor dietary ailments such as constipation, indigestion and common food allergies.

All this is relevant to your tiny baby as the damage can start early. The early signs of fatal heart disease, such as arterial plaque and fatty streaks in the arteries, can be found as early as one–two years of age. The blood pressure of children under ten in developed Western societies is significantly higher than those in traditional non-Western societies. Autopsies on children as young as eight years old already show evidence of the early stages of heart disease. The good news is that studies with young children have shown that a change in diet which cuts down on saturated fats and increases fibre, protein and carbohydrate intake can significantly reduce cholesterol levels, even over relatively quite short periods. This is especially noteworthy for those who come from families with histories of heart disease or high heart disease risk factors.

Tooth decay must be the most prevalent disorder in our society. Half of our children suffer tooth decay in their first teeth. A staggering 90 percent of the population will suffer from tooth decay in their second teeth while still in their teens.

Changes in the way the dental service is funded means that a poor diet will not only hurt the oral health of you child, but also your purse. Directly relevant to dental health are the inappropriately called 'baby drinks' (more about these on page 91–3). It is also shocking how many babies are given sweets and confectionery at a very early age. From a government survey of the diets of six- to twelve-month-old babies it was found than 63 percent were given cakes, buns and puddings, 67 percent were fed sweet biscuits and 45 percent ate chocolate confectionery. The entire British population spent £4.4 billion on confectionery last year – an average of £76 per person. This means that there is an average of 1/2lb of confectionery consumed each week by each person. No wonder the British nation has such a history of tooth decay.

Diet and Development

Good nutrition is essential for the development of every child. Children who do not obtain the essential vitamins and minerals from their diets do not grow as much in comparison to other children. They also suffer more frequently from infections and lose valuable time from school.

There is also evidence that diet affects mental as well as physical development. Studies into this possible link began back in the 1960s. One study divided students into high and low vitamin C groups. There was an extraordinary difference of 4.5 IQ points between the average IQ for each group. In Massachusetts, researchers have concluded that the more refined foods we eat the less intelligent we are. This result was reached after correlating the increasing proportion of the diet made up of refined carbohydrates (such as sugar, commercial cereals, white bread and sweets), with decreasing IQ levels. The IQ score varied by a staggering 25 points. Studies have also been

BABY AND TODDLER FOOD

carried out where schoolchildren have been given vitamin supplements. These studies have the advantage of an effective control group – unknown to the children some were given vitamins and others a placebo or dummy pill. Many such studies have shown a significant improvement in the IQ levels (such as 10–15 points or more) of the children taking the vitamin supplements, while there is no change in the control group. Given that one in five children suffers from learning difficulties, these findings are significant for the future intelligence of the nation. Interestingly, children who are autistic appear to respond even more to 'nutrition therapy' and more research is clearly needed in this important area.

Appoint yourself as Health Engineer

You decide everything for your child: it is only fair – given the far-reaching consequences – to provide the best diet possible. Giving a nutritious balanced diet does not mean an expensive outlay. In fact, it can be cheaper than a diet that consists largely of expensive commercial baby food. As a general rule, a baby or toddler can eat a small amount of the food you give to the rest of the family, which allows you to take advantage of bulk buying and reduces preparation time. You also lose nothing on the taste front either. Healthy food is probably amongst the tastiest there is and has a far more natural taste than commercial foods which need additives to make them palatable.

As a baby and then a toddler, your child is growing and developing at an amazing rate. It is also the time of life when a person is learning at their fastest rate. You could say foundations are being laid – and you would not expect a house built on poor foundations to stand for very long. So appoint yourself as a responsible engineer of your child's future health. Your child's health and well-being is simply too important to ignore.

2
A Child's Nutrition

It is important and relevant for us all to understand the basics of nutrition. The big building blocks are the macronutrients – proteins, carbohydrates and fats. Equally necessary are the tiny blocks of the micronutrients – vitamins and minerals. More important for life than food is water; a human being can last for quite a while without food but for only a few days without water. These six elements are the essentials for a healthy life.

An easy way to remember the basics of a nutritious diet is to follow this healthy eating pyramid (see below). Eat most of the

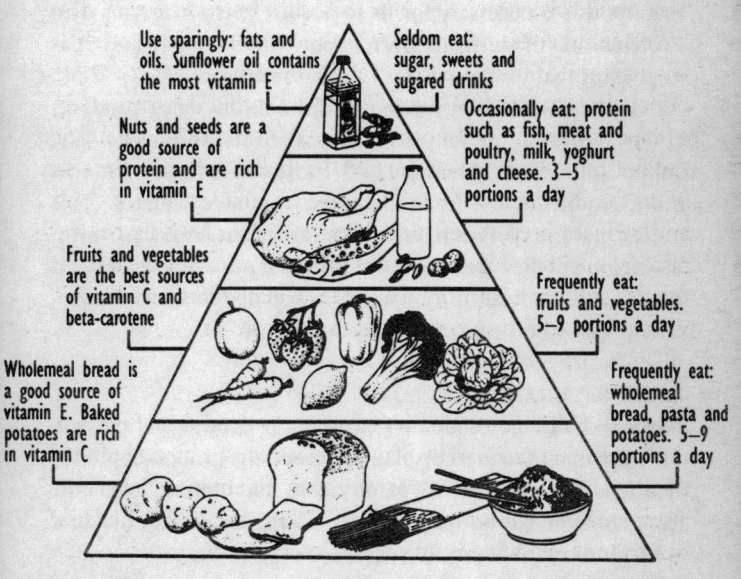

Use sparingly: fats and oils. Sunflower oil contains the most vitamin E

Seldom eat: sugar, sweets and sugared drinks

Nuts and seeds are a good source of protein and are rich in vitamin E

Occasionally eat: protein such as fish, meat and poultry, milk, yoghurt and cheese. 3–5 portions a day

Fruits and vegetables are the best sources of vitamin C and beta-carotene

Frequently eat: fruits and vegetables. 5–9 portions a day

Wholemeal bread is a good source of vitamin E. Baked potatoes are rich in vitamin C

Frequently eat: wholemeal bread, pasta and potatoes. 5–9 portions a day

BABY AND TODDLER FOOD

foods in the bottom layers and little (or even none) of some of the foods in the top layers. A diet composed in this way will provide you with the correct proportion of macronutrients and a healthy dose of the micronutrients.

The Macronutrients

PROTEIN

The word 'protein' is derived from the Greek meaning basic or fundamental, and proteins are fundamental to all living matter. In humans, protein accounts for 17 percent of our total body mass. Proteins are used for the growth and repair of our bodies, being required for these purposes by each individual cell. Any extra can be stored and used later as a source of energy. Some proteins are termed 'essential' as our bodies cannot synthesise them and it is necessary for us to acquire them from our diet. Proteins are made from over twenty amino acids and it is important that we receive our full share of these.

Good sources of protein are fish, meat, dairy produce, grains, pulses (especially soya beans), nuts and seeds. The animal sources of protein are both more concentrated and in a more readily usable form than the vegetable sources. This means that vegetarians have to take care to eat enough protein, but as long as they are aware of this need it poses no problem. It is also perfectly healthy to bring up babies and toddlers as vegetarians (see The Vegetarian Baby on page 86–7).

CARBOHYDRATE

Carbohydrates are made up of carbon, hydrogen and oxygen. They are manufactured by plants through the process of photosynthesis. This is when the plant makes starch using the energy from sunlight. Carbohydrates form a large part of our diet and are an important source of energy.

A CHILD'S NUTRITION

There is a whole spectrum of differently sized molecules within the carbohydrates. The size of molecule provides a rough guide to the value of that type of carbohydrate in terms of nutrition – the larger the molecule the better the carbohydrate is for us. This is because the larger molecules are found in complex carbohydrates, which release their energy gradually. Complex carbohydrates are such foods as potatoes, pasta, grains and bread which should make up the majority of our diet, (see the Healthy Eating Pyramid on page 9). The smaller molecules are sugars which release their energy very swiftly into the blood. Although this can provide a pick-me-up, it is very short-lived and is rapidly followed by a blood-sugar low, which makes us feel tired, lethargic and can even cause headaches. This sugar 'low' also creates a craving for more sugar which, if indulged in, can result in a sugar cycle of cravings, energy bursts and depressing lows. This leads to many health problems and weight gain.

When talking about sugar, it is important to draw a distinction between extrinsic and intrinsic sugar. Intrinsic sugar is that naturally found in a food, such as fructose in fruit and lactose in milk. Extrinsic sugar is that which is added to food and it is this sugar which is not only bad for us but also totally unnecessary. If someone (including your toddler) does have a sugar craving, try to satisfy it with some fruit – white grapes are especially good, being a fun snack to eat and more than sweet enough. The advantage of the intrinsic sugar, fructose, in the fruit does not mean 'empty calories' as your child is also getting a healthy dose of vitamins and dietary fibre.

The largest size of carbohydrate molecule is found in cellulose, more commonly known as dietary fibre, which is indigestible. Although this does not provide nutrition as it cannot be absorbed, it is essential for keeping our digestive systems operating effectively and healthily.

The other vitally important point to be made about carbohydrates is the distinction between refined and unrefined carbohydrates. The unrefined and more natural forms are definitely the healthier alternatives. The refined forms have often been stripped of most if not all of their vitamins and minerals and a large proportion of dietary fibre. It is very easy to make the change from refined to unrefined versions and this simple switch can improve everyone's diet – from babies and beyond.

Table 1
Refined versus unrefined foods

REFINED = LESS HEALTHY	UNREFINED = MORE HEALTHY
Sugars: Sugar (including anything made with sugar, eg biscuits, cakes, jellies, soft drinks, etc.) Sweets Honey	**Sugars:** Fruit Vegetables Juices (fruit/vegetable) Puddings and biscuits, etc. made with the sugars found in fruit
Complex carbohydrates: White flour, bread and pasta White rice Processed breakfast cereals (although some are better than others – see page 63–5)	**Complex carbohydrates:** Brown flour, bread and pasta Brown rice (brown is beautiful!) Whole-grain breakfast cereals Potatoes Pulses

FATS

Fat is a necessary component of our bodies. Fat keeps us warm, is a store of energy, keeps our skin and arteries supple, protects our internal organs and is essential for proper brain function. In a normal man it accounts for about 12 percent of the total body weight and in a woman about 25 percent.

But fat has had a very bad press in recent years. This is slightly misleading as we do actually need to eat some fat. However, most of us eat too much fat, particularly fat of the wrong sort. Recommendations are that we get no more than 30 percent of all our calories from fat, but the average intake is around 45 percent. More significant is the *type* of fat we eat. There are two main types – saturated and unsaturated.

Saturated fats are really only useful as a source of energy and padding, and can contribute to harmful high cholesterol levels and to coronary disease later in life. As adults we obtain enough energy from other sources so it is totally unnecessary to eat saturated fat – cut saturated fat out of your diet as much as possible. This villain is found in animal produce, particularly in red meat, cheese, butter, full-fat milk, eggs and much fast food. It is very simple to cut down the amount of saturated fat by trimming all the visible fat and skin off meat, by switching to skimmed or semi-skimmed milk and always cooking with vegetable oil instead of butter or lard.

It is important to note that once small children start to drink cows' milk they should be given full-fat milk until they are at least two years' old, and generally until they are slightly older. For a while after weaning, milk should remain a principal food in their diets. This is because they need the fat as a source of energy for their swiftly growing and active young bodies. Babies on a milk-only diet obtain 54 percent of their energy from fat, whereas in a healthy adult diet less than 30 percent of energy should be obtained from fat. The change in the composition of diet should happen very gradually. For all other sources of saturated fats apart from milk – what goes for adults goes for kids too: cut them out of the diet!

Unsaturated fats on the other hand are derived from vegetable sources. These fats are generally liquid at room temperatures, and so are called oils. Chemically speaking, an oil is exactly the same as a fat. As well as providing the all-important essential fatty acids, dietary fats are often carriers of the fat-soluble vitamins A, D, E and K. Use a vegetable oil such as olive oil when cooking in place of butter or other saturated fats. When buying your vegetable oils make sure you buy cold-pressed, unrefined oils as these also contain the highest levels of nutrients (refined versions look paler as they have been largely stripped of their nutrients). Another excellent source of unsaturated fat, packed full of goodness, is any oily fish, such as salmon and mackerel.

Table 2
Saturated versus unsaturated fats

Saturated = Less healthy	Unsaturated = More healthy
Meat fat	Vegetable oils (eg olive, safflower, sesame, sunflower, soya and walnut oils)
Lard, suet or dripping	
Whole milk, butter, cheese and full-fat yoghurt	Fish oils (eg in mackerel, herrings and sardines)
Egg yolks	

The Micronutrients

VITAMINS

Vitamins are essential for complete health. The human body is unable to manufacture them (with the sole exception of vitamin D produced in the skin in the presence of sunlight) so they must be obtained from the food we eat. Diets lacking in particular vitamins may produce vitamin deficiency diseases, including scurvy, beriberi and rickets. However, they are not needed simply to prevent these diseases but also for the efficient day-to-day running of the complex machine of the human body. Recent research has started to show that vitamins have an amazing impact on our health. Many of us, however, do not receive the levels of vitamins necessary for this optimum nutrition. If your children follow the Healthy Eating Pyramid on page 9 they will receive a good input of vitamins. As even this may not be sufficient, especially with the destruction of vitamins in foods through storage and processing methods and the increased needs of our bodies caused by today's pollution and stressful living, it is recommended that we all take a good multi-vitamin and mineral supplement. The government recommends that all babies and toddlers are given children's vitamin drops every day from the age of six months until they are at least two years' old and preferably until five years' old. These contain vitamins A, C and D, and are available from chemists, or at a lower cost from your child-health clinic. As children grow older it should be noted that their vitamin requirements increase, so again a multi-vitamin and mineral supplement may be beneficial. Remember to check that the supplement is suitable for children, as they should not be given adult dosages.

In the following table of Vitamins, the nutrients have been divided into fat- or water-soluble vitamins. The body is able to store the fat-soluble vitamins, and so long as the body receives enough it can regulate its own supply and demand. The body is unable to store the water-soluble vitamins, so any excess to demand is excreted from the body in urine. Therefore, it is necessary to keep the supply of these vitamins fairly constant to avoid shortages.

Table 3
Vitamins

Vitamin	Needed for	Good sources
Fat soluble:		
A	growth, healthy skin, lungs, good night vision	healthy orange/red/dark green fruit and vegetables (eg carrots, tomatoes, sweet potatoes, apricots, peaches, broccoli, watercress), oily fish, liver, eggs (Beta carotene is a form of vitamin A which acts as an antioxidant destroying free radicals, and this is found in colourful fruit and vegetables.)
D	bone formation and health (it works in conjunction with calcium)	fish, liver, eggs; the majority of our requirements are fulfilled by the vitamin D produced by the skin in the presence of sunlight.

A CHILD'S NUTRITION

Vitamin	Needed for	Good sources
E	maintaining healthy cell structure, good circulation and maintaining red blood cells; an antioxidant	vegetable oils, nuts, seeds, whole grains, avocados
K	blood clotting and bone maintenance	present in our intestines, found in most vegetables and whole-grain cereals

Water soluble:

C	strengthening the immune system, helping fight infection, aiding growth of healthy tissue; an antioxidant	fruit (especially citrus fruits, melons, strawberries and tomatoes), vegetables (especially potatoes, broccoli, spinach and cauliflower)
B complex (there are many B vitamins)	growth, healthy nervous system, aid to digestion, converting food into energy	liver, yeast extract, fish, meat, dairy produce, whole-grain cereals, nuts, potatoes, dark green vegetables, bananas

MINERALS

Around 6 percent of our body weight is made up of minerals. Calcium, phosphorus and magnesium are the principal constituents of our bones. Other minerals, vital for life, are used to regulate and balance our body chemistry. It is important that your child does not become deficient in calcium (another very good reason why milk should remain a major food even after weaning) or iron. Calcium is needed for the swiftly developing bones of young children. If cow's milk cannot be given due to an allergy, calcium-enriched varieties of soya milk should be substituted (normal soya milk contains little calcium). However, these can be very high in sugar, so consult your doctor first. Iron is needed for physical and mental development — a deficiency can delay this development and lead to behavioural changes. Iron deficiency is the most prevalent single nutrient deficiency in the world, affecting one billion people — one-fifth of the world's population. Infants are the most susceptible group due to high demands for growth coupled with a diet often low in easily absorbable sources of iron.

Chromium, copper, manganese, selenium and zinc are known as the 'trace' minerals — they are all essential for us to remain healthy but we only require them in tiny amounts.

Water

The spring of life — water is essential for us all to live. About 60 percent of the human body is made up of water. We lose water through excretion, perspiration and exhalation, and this water is replaced through drinking and eating. Feeling thirsty is a rough guideline to when we need more water, but if you feel thirsty your body dehydrated around twenty minutes ago! It is therefore important to drink fluids even when you do not feel

Table 4
Minerals

Mineral	Needed for	Good sources
Calcium	strong, healthy bones (especially in childhood), good teeth, efficient muscle working	dairy produce, especially milk, fruit, broccoli, pulses
Iron	healthy blood (iron is a vital component of haemoglobin which transports oxygen around the body) and muscles	liver, red meat, oily fish, egg yolks, dried fruits (especially apricots), whole grains, lentils, baked beans, green leafy vegetables
Magnesium	healthy bones and muscles (works with calcium), protein and hormone organisation	green leafy vegetables, nuts, seeds
Potassium	nerve transmission, water balance	fruit, vegetables, whole grains
Sodium	nerve transmission, water balance	salt – but we do not need to add any extra sodium (salt) as it is present in most foods in small amounts

BABY AND TODDLER FOOD

thirsty and to offer children plenty of water. A baby generally obtains all the water it needs through breast or formula milk, but in very hot weather this can be supplemented with cooled, boiled water. Even after weaning the best drinks for a small child are milk or water. An alternative is diluted fruit juice which also contains useful vitamins. Beware of commercial baby drinks and other drinks and squashes which are high in sugar and additives (see pages 91–3).

The Villains

The six dietary sins for babies and toddlers are: *salt, saturated fat, sugar, chemical additives, alcohol, caffeine*

SALT
This should never be added to a baby's or a toddler's food. Their smaller body systems cannot cope with more salt than is found naturally in foods. Remember to watch out for added salt when giving them the same food as the rest of the family. In fact, it wouldn't do the adults any harm to cut down on salt too as an excess of salt overloads the kidneys and causes water retention. At present the average adult daily intake is 12g daily, whereas the World Health Organisation recommends no more than 5g daily.

SATURATED FAT
Our diet as a nation contains far too much saturated fat. Eating an excess is one of the main causes of our biggest killer – heart disease. It also leads to an increased risk of cancer. In the shorter term it means we put on weight and our lymphatic system slows down. We can cut out saturated fats with relative ease and replace them with unsaturated fats. Apart from full-fat milk, once over a year old, you should not give your baby or toddler many foods high in saturated fat.

A CHILD'S NUTRITION

SUGAR

Too much sugar makes us put on weight, which leads to high blood pressure, strokes and heart disease. It has also been linked to lowered immunity, kidney disorders, diabetes and some skin disorders. A high-sugar diet can also trigger hyperactivity and there is an unequivocal link between sugar and tooth decay. To give babies a diet high in sugar is to set these things in motion, as well as giving them a sweet tooth which may lead to a high sugar diet throughout life. It is important never to create an association of sweets or sweet foods with rewards. Instead of sweets, how about a handful of dried fruit or a piece of exotic fruit? Or try rewarding with a small present – such as a small toy, a comic or balloon, or a special trip or outing. Beware of commercially produced baby foods which often contain vast amounts of sugar, sometimes in spite of being marketed as healthy. Prime examples of this are breakfast cereals and fruit drinks.

CHEMICAL ADDITIVES

Added to many processed foods to give them the 'right' taste, texture and colour. Some of these have been banned in foods specifically for small children, but can often lurk in family foods bought for tiny tots. Get to grips with E-numbers and read the labels before you buy. See *Reading the Labels* on pp.94–8 and the quick-reference *Additive Decoder* on pp.98–106.

ALCOHOL

Of course we don't give children alcoholic drinks, but alcohol can crop up in other forms. Check that the gripe water you give your baby does not contain alcohol and watch out for puddings such as sherry trifle. Even small amounts of alcohol can be damaging to a baby's kidneys and digestive system. Be particularly careful not to drink alcohol when breast feeding. Never be tempted to give a small child sips of your own alcoholic drinks. Just one glass of spirits can kill a toddler.

BABY AND TODDLER FOOD

CAFFEINE

All cola drinks contain the artificial stimulant caffeine. These should not be given to small children as caffeine can disrupt their nervous system. Fizzy drinks also contain phosphates which prevent the absorption of valuable calcium into growing bones. Avoid giving tea and coffee to small children as these are diuretic and will encourage fluid loss. Tea and coffee can over-stimulate children, leading to disruptive behaviour and sleepless nights.

In addition to the above, some other foods should be avoided until your baby is a certain age, mainly because eating some foods too early seems to lead to food intolerance and allergies. This aspect is covered in more detail in Chapter 5; in particular, see the *What When Weaning* table on pages 42–3 which shows what foods can be given and when.

Table 5
Minimum Nutritional Requirements

	Less than 1 year	1-2 years	2-3 years
Calories (Kcal)	800	1,200-1,400	1,600
Protein (g)	20	30-35	40
Calcium (mg)	600	500-600	500-600
Phosphorus (mg)	150	400	500
Potassium (mg)	500	1,000	1,250
Magnesium (mg)	40	100	125
Iron (mg)	6	7	8
Vitamin A (mcg)	450	300	300
Vitamin B1 (mg)	0.3	0.5	0.6
Vitamin B2 (mg)	0.4	0.7	0.8
Vitamin B6 (mg)	0.4	0.7	1.0
Vitamin B12 (mcg)	2	3	3
Nicotinic acid (mg)	5	8	9
Folic acid (mg)	0.1	0.2	0.2
Pantothenic acid (mg)	2	3	4
Vitamin C (mg)	15	20	20
Vitamin D (mg)	10	10	10
Vitamin E (mcg)	5	8	10

3
What to Give When

In this chapter we will look at what foods you should give your child and when. There are also plenty of tips on how to encourage children to grow up eating healthily and enjoying their food. This guidance is important as babies are born with two conflicting eating habits. Babies can regulate their total intake of calories by refusing milk once the correct amount has been obtained. However, on the other hand, a baby is also born with an innate preference for sweet (and highly calorific) foods. At the end of this chapter there is a *What When Weaning* table for easy at-a-glance reference. It tells you when foods should be introduced and which foods should be avoided at what ages.

The Newborn Baby

In the first few months of life a baby's nutritional requirements are completely fulfilled by a single food – milk. This is either breast or formula milk; a baby should not be given cows' milk until over a year old as this does not contain enough nutrients for healthy growth.

Breast is Best

Breast milk is the most natural food for your baby and there are many very good reasons why breast is best:
* Breast milk is designed specifically to feed your baby and it contains all the nutrients needed in the correct

BABY AND TODDLER FOOD

proportions. However closely formula milk mimics breast milk, it is very much the poor relation. Formula milk does not contain many of the important constituents of breast milk such as selenium and the essential fatty acids GLA, DHA and EPA, nor does it contain antibodies for disease prevention or active human growth hormones for healthy development.

* To meet the needs of the baby precisely, breast milk actually varies in composition at differing times after the birth, during the day and even within a single feed.
* Easily digested, breast milk is less likely to cause stomach upsets, diarrhoea or constipation.
* The antibodies found in milk help protect against infections. A bottle-fed baby is twice as likely to get a cold and four times as likely to catch pneumonia.
* It has been medically proven that breast-fed babies are less likely to develop certain diseases later in life. Breast-fed babies have even been found to be marginally more intelligent and to have a higher IQ rating, possibly due to the presence in breast milk of unique essential fatty acids needed for brain development.
* There is also evidence that breast feeding can help prevent some allergies, or at least lessen the severity. If your family has a history of allergies, eczema or asthma this may be particularly relevant.
* Breast milk is the ultimate in practicality – always ready when needed, at the correct temperature and requiring no sterilising.
* Formula milks are expensive – breast milk is free!
* Breast feeding helps develop a special relationship between mother and baby, and can be a real pleasure.

The government's *Health of the Nation* Green Paper aims to have 75 percent of all new mothers breast feeding by the year 2000.

Problems?

Breast feeding is not without its difficulties, but these are almost always surmountable hurdles. If you do encounter problems, hold on to the fact that it really is the best option for your baby and worth persevering with. Contact your local branch of the National Childbirth Trust or La Leche League (a breast-feeding support network) who are both sympathetic and helpful; their local telephone numbers will be in the phone book. These organisations have experienced counsellors on call and can also arrange the hire of useful equipment such as electric breast pumps. It is worth remembering that if timing in relation to other commitments or work is the problem, you can keep expressed milk in bottles in the fridge (it also freezes well). Ameda have a mail-order service for many useful breast-feeding accessories. Details of all these organisations are in *Useful Addresses* at the end of this book.

Breast milk works on a simple supply and demand principle. So the more the baby feeds the more milk is produced. An exception to this is if the baby is not sucking efficiently. If this is the case, ask your midwife or health visitor for advice. To suck properly, the baby needs to feed with a wide-open mouth, taking in the nipple and much of the coloured area around (the areola). To achieve this, hold the baby close to you with his chest (not side) turned towards you. Once the baby is 'latched on' his chin should be touching your breast. If the baby is sucking at the nipple only, not much milk will be obtained and your baby is likely to be dissatisfied soon after finishing the feed.

If the baby is not sucking properly it can lead to other problems, one of which is sore nipples – try different feeding positions and they should improve. In the meantime, a thick nipple cream such as those containing natural chamomile or calendula extracts will help relieve the soreness. If your breasts feel tender, lumpy or swollen, take some milk off straight away either by putting the baby to the breast or by expressing some milk by

BABY AND TODDLER FOOD

hand. Leaving the breasts full of milk can lead to a blocked milk duct and then a painful breast infection, called mastitis. This will make you feel feverish, tired and aching, with headaches. The breasts themselves can become inflamed, sore to touch and may show red patches. The best way to treat this condition is to feed often (which is also the best preventative measure). Try different positions as the blockage could be caused by bad positioning – such as being hunched over your baby or the baby sucking on the end of the nipple. To ease the discomfort, try sponging your breasts with warm water or applying hot flannels to unblock the ducts.

It is essential to adopt a good breast-feeding position. You must be comfortable and able to hold the baby for quite a while without strain. Try experimenting with different chairs and positions, or even lying down on your side with the baby up against you. A pillow to help support the baby can also help make life more comfortable.

Being comfortable and relaxed is important for the 'let-down' reflex. This is the reflex which literally lets down the milk so it gathers behind the nipple and surrounding area. It will generally occur when the baby starts sucking but can happen even before you start feeding. In the early weeks your breasts may even leak milk as you think of your baby. This reflex is very necessary as otherwise your baby cannot reach your milk. However, for this reflex to work fully you do need to be fairly relaxed – it can be hindered by stress, worry, exhaustion or perhaps embarrassment. Soothing music, or burning some sweet-scented essential oils in a diffuser, may help you to relax.

It is important to take care of yourself when breast feeding as you will produce less milk when tired or low in energy. Eat a nutritious balanced diet – it may be helpful to eat smaller amounts at regular intervals to keep your energy levels high. Everything you eat will be passed to your offspring, so eat well. Remember that the caffeine in tea, coffee and cola is likely to

WHAT TO GIVE WHEN

keep your baby awake. Do not smoke while breast feeding as the poisons will pass straight through into your breast milk. Also remember to drink plenty of liquids, as you need to keep replacing the fluid lost through milk production. Try and stay rested – not easy with a small baby and even harder if there are other older children! However, take advantage of the times the baby sleeps – maybe take a catnap yourself, put your feet up and read or listen to music, or pamper yourself with a relaxing bath or a bit of self-massage – the chores can wait! These moments are a very special time just for you and will help you to retain your separate identity so you don't feel that you exist simply as your baby's milking machine.

Some babies settle into a feeding pattern quite quickly. Others do not, but this is nothing to worry about. Feed when your baby asks to be fed and let the feed go on until the baby wants to stop. Those who start limiting the length or frequency of feeds are firstly in danger of getting blocked milk ducts and secondly likely to lessen and then stop their milk supply. When feeding, do not swap the baby from one breast to another until the sucking stops voluntarily. This is to allow the more nourishing hindmilk which comes later in the feed to be reached. The foremilk which is less nourishing is more of a thirst quencher before the serious business starts. And last but definitely not least – *enjoy* breast feeding your baby!

Formula milk

Although breast is undoubtedly best, it is not always possible for a mother to breast feed. Feeding problems do put many new mothers off the idea and breast feeding can also be difficult while working. If you do decide not to breast feed, you must feed your baby on a special formula milk as these contain a suitable ratio of nutrients for infants and are quite easily digested. Despite the glossy advertising campaigns, there is not much difference between the brands. As a leading paediatrician (who

BABY AND TODDLER FOOD

prefers to remain unnamed) puts it: 'Do you really believe there is a difference between types of petrol? The same is true of baby milks. Your choice solely depends on whom you want to give your money to.'

To make up feeds, follow the instructions on the container. It is important to follow the directions on how much water to add to how much powder. Remember to use cooled, boiled water to make up the feeds. I prefer to filter my tap-water in a filter-jug to screen out many of its less desirable components, such as chlorine, lead and nitrates. You may find it convenient to make up a day's feeds at a time and store the bottles in the fridge. Never keep a made-up feed for more than twenty-four hours.

It is always important to sterilise all the equipment before using as dirty bottles and teats are the perfect breeding ground for germs. Sterilising can be done by boiling, steaming or chemical methods. Always clean all the equipment in a weak solution of washing-up liquid and scrub with a bottle brush before sterilising. For steaming, use a special steam sterilising unit available from all good baby shops. Follow the instructions that come with this type of steriliser carefully. For chemical sterilisation, you will have to immerse all the equipment in a sterilising solution – don't forget the teats and bottle tops. Tablets to make up such a solution are readily available from chemists and baby-equipment shops, and are useful when travelling. The cheapest method of sterilisation is boiling. Simply place all the equipment in a large pan of water making sure there is no air trapped in the bottles, cover with a lid and boil for ten minutes. Leave to cool before using.

Four–Six Months – Introducing Solids

The majority of babies receive their first mouthfuls of so-called solids between the ages of four and six months. Few babies

WHAT TO GIVE WHEN

should be given solids before the age of three months, as a young baby's digestive system is not capable of absorbing foods more complex than baby milk. It is now generally accepted that the longer you leave the introduction of solids the better (this is relatively recent thinking) to avoid the early introduction of certain foods linked to allergy problems and food intolerances. In America, some paediatricians suggest that solid foods are not given until a baby is six months' old. However, it is important that all babies receive some solid food by or soon after six months, as by then the iron reserves that they are born with will have run out.

Remember that each baby is an individual and so no hard and fast rule can be made about the 'right' age to start eating solids. Let your baby tell you when he or she is ready to eat solids. Try giving solids when:

* your baby is still hungry after a good milk feed (eg 225ml, 8fl oz)
* feeds become more frequent over a prolonged period
* your baby appears more restless than normal, especially at night.

WHAT TO GIVE

It is important to remember that the primary source of nutrition at this stage is still milk. The amount of milk given should therefore not be reduced – the initial solids are in addition to the milk. The best food to begin with is a thin porridge made from oat flakes, rice flakes or cornmeal, and a little breast or formula milk (see the *What Weaning When* table on pages 42–3). Commercial baby rice (plain) is excellent as a starter food. It has the great advantage of extreme convenience and most brands are nutritionally sound. Check that the baby rice you buy is completely salt and sugar free. Now is an excellent time to get into the habit of reading *all* the labels when buying baby foods. Many unwanted added extras can lurk in processed

BABY AND TODDLER FOOD

foods, so it is always worth a glance to check (see *Reading the Labels* on pp. 94–8).

Begin to introduce new flavours after a couple of weeks. It is best to leave a few days in between each new flavour as taste is a new experience to a baby and it is better not to overwhelm tiny taste buds. This also gives you an opportunity to watch for any allergic reaction, such as diarrhoea or skin rashes. The ideal foods are puréed fruit and vegetables, which are an excellent way of giving your baby a good supply of vital vitamins and minerals. Good ones to try are apple, pear, banana, carrot, parsnip, broccoli, spinach and sweet potato. If your baby refuses a food, don't try and force the issue, just take it away and try again a couple of weeks later – you may find it becomes a favourite second time around. To make a purée cook the fruit or vegetable until it is soft and then thoroughly mash with a fork. It is a good idea to use a blender or push the food through a sieve to achieve a smooth consistency.

WHAT NOT TO GIVE

Small babies should not be given any salt, sugar or fatty foods. At this stage you should also avoid the following: Milk apart from breast or formula milk (so cows' milk is out), all other dairy products including cheese, eggs, wheat-based foods (such as wheat cereals and pasta, citrus fruits and summer fruits (such as strawberries and raspberries). The reason for avoiding these foods is because they may lead to allergic reactions, so they are better left until your baby is a few months older. Other foods to avoid are tomatoes, which are highly acidic, and spices, chillies and nuts.

SOLID SUGGESTIONS

* Offer the solid food on a small, shallow plastic teaspoon or on the tip of a clean finger.
* Offer food in the middle or at the end of a milk feed as

WHAT TO GIVE WHEN

your baby will be more receptive to the idea once the initial hunger pangs have been satisfied.

* Many people also find their babies to be more receptive if they remain in the feeding position and relax – don't tense up or make a big issue out of food.
* It is a good idea to make the 'solid' food fairly wet and soft to begin with, maybe even adding some breast or formula milk, unsweetened fruit juice or cooled, boiled water. As your baby gets more accustomed to solid food you can make the purées thicker and slightly coarser in texture.
* Be prepared for a mess! Have plenty of wipes, a bib and muslin cloth handy.
* Don't expect your baby to eat masses of food, just one–two teaspoons once a day is plenty for first feeds. Gradually increase the amount of food on demand. Build up slowly to giving solids at three feeds a day, but be guided by your own baby's appetite.
* To save time, it is easier to make a whole batch of a purée and freeze it in small quantities. Try using a plastic ice-cube tray to freeze small meal-sized portions.

COMMERCIAL BABY FOODS

It is frequently better and generally more nutritious to give your baby home-made foods cooked from fresh ingredients. However, it is sometimes more convenient, especially when travelling, to take a jar of commercial baby food. It saves on mess and the one thing you can be certain of with these baby foods is the hygiene and convenience factor. Always read the label before buying (see *Reading the Labels* on pages 94–8) and do not be misled by the advertising hype and exaggerated label claims. Just because the food you cook doesn't have a nutrition table stamped on the side doesn't mean that it is not packed full of goodness. In fact, home-made foods without such labels are

BABY AND TODDLER FOOD

more often than not healthier as they are made with fresh ingredients and contain fewer additives, such as preservatives and starchy bulking agents.

DRINKS

Babies usually obtain sufficient fluids from their formula or breast milk. If your baby is still thirsty after a feed offer only cooled, boiled water.

Six–Nine Months – Variety is the Spice of Life

Researchers have noted that children between the ages of six and eighteen months are more receptive to new tastes than at any other time in their lives. So now is the time to introduce all sorts of new foods and exciting flavours. This is a golden opportunity to give babies many different types of fresh fruit and vegetables to ensure they will grow up willing to eat their greens. Researchers have also noticed that in babies and small children there is a direct relationship between the number of times a child is presented with a specific food and a preference for that food, so give foods you want your child to like regularly. Now is also a good time for new foods as this is when milk teeth begin to appear and a baby is open to a variety of coarser textures and the notion of chewing.

Don't ever force food on a baby. If your child does not want a particular food, follow the same rule as before – take it away and try again in a few weeks' time. If your baby only wants a tiny bit of solid food, that is fine, although some babies like their food so much that they cry between mouthfuls. (This is often due to the frustration of food arriving in fits and starts instead of a continuous stream.) Always be guided by your child's personal preference and never make feeding time a battle ground. All babies will eat when they are hungry!

WHAT TO GIVE WHEN

WHAT TO GIVE

As well as the fruit, vegetables and porridges you were giving previously you can also introduce proteins such as plain yoghurt, pulses, white fish, well-cooked chicken and egg yolks. At this stage the food should still be of a mushy consistency, so foods should be puréed until relatively smooth, although slightly coarser than before. Wheat-based products can also be given, so you can actually start giving adult breakfast cereals such as Weetabix or Ready Brek – although check the label as some breakfast cereals are ridiculously high in sugar. Your baby might also enjoy investigating the wide choice of grains such as millet flakes, barley flakes, quinoa and oatmeal which all make excellent baby foods and are readily available from health-food shops. A wider variety of fruit and vegetables can now be offered raw, including carrot sticks and celery stalks to chew on. Take advantage of nature's convenience foods when travelling and unzip a banana or split a ripe pear in two and scoop out the delicious inside.

Remember to keep up the formula or breast milk feeds. Again, follow what your baby dictates; if he or she is eating plenty of solid food then slightly less milk can be given. However, a baby who does not eat many solids still requires the nutrition and energy provided by the milk feeds. All children should drink at least a pint of milk every day until at least two years' old and, ideally, for several more years. Some nutritionists recommend this amount of milk until five years of age. (*Note:* Cows' milk can be given after the first year.) There is no need to give older babies 'follow-on' formula milks if they are eating a well-balanced diet. These formula milks for older babies are an unnecessary expense and a bore to prepare.

The other main nutrient likely to be lacking in a baby's diet is iron. All babies are born with a good supply of iron and when this is added to the iron they automatically receive from breast milk or formula feeds the supply will last until they are five or

BABY AND TODDLER FOOD

six months' old. After this time, babies need to be given foods containing iron, for example sieved green vegetables such as broccoli and spinach or well-cooked egg yolks.

What not to give

Continue to avoid the terrible trio of salt, sugar and fatty foods. It is still advisable to steer clear of cows' milk and other dairy products, although in small amounts they are fine, for instance if used when cooking food for the whole family. Also on the no-no list are egg whites, nuts, spices and chillies because these can often cause an allergic reaction.

Teething tips

By now your baby will be grabbing all sorts of things – and straight in the mouth they go. This is another opportunity for new tastes – all babies enjoy something more than a tasteless plastic ring on which to cut their gums.

* Slow-bake some bread until really hard, then cut into easily held sticks. A quicker alternative is a crust of toast, although this is more likely to disintegrate when chewed.
* Half a peeled carrot is good and hard for teething gums.
* Very few babies dislike fruit – slices of peeled apple work a treat.
* Rusks are the traditional teething food but beware as some of these (even the 'low sugar' ones) can contain more sugar than pieces of confectionery, and they all contain some sugar – so always check the labels. Babies don't need biscuits for energy.
* Never leave a baby unattended when eating as they could swallow unchewed pieces of food and choke. If your baby does try to swallow too large a piece, take it

out with a bent finger. If this doesn't work, place the infant face-down across your lap and pat firmly on the upper back.

DRINKS

Between six and nine months your baby will probably still not need any other drinks apart from breast or formula milk, and the best alternative if your baby is thirsty continues to be cooled, boiled water. However, if you have started to cut down the milk feeds because your baby is eating a lot of solids, you may want to offer water a little more regularly. Alternatively, use pure fruit juice, such as apple juice, well diluted with cooled, boiled water – one part of juice to three or four parts of water. This is a good occasional drink and it is naturally sweet. Do not give a baby commercial drinks which are packed full of added sugar – not only are these expensive, they can also encourage a taste for high-sugar flavours.

Nine–Twelve Months – The Age of Patience

This is the time your baby really begins to experiment at mealtimes. Not only through the new tastes and textures which you continue to give, but also in the method of feeding. At this time, babies begin to learn to do things for themselves and may well start trying to grab the food. In this event, finger foods are an excellent idea (see page 37). However, most of a baby's foods will still need to be eaten with a spoon. Try holding the spoon at the end so that your baby can hold the handle further up, then guide both the hand and spoon so that the food goes on target for the mouth. In a relatively short time your baby will probably learn to get the spoon to his mouth himself. Your baby may also enjoy experimenting with a teaching beaker and should definitely be encouraged to hold his own bottle.

BABY AND TODDLER FOOD

Many books advocate giving your child the spoon and letting the food fly. This attitude has its advantages as it allows your child to experiment and enjoy food, but it also has a huge downside. It does not necessarily encourage your child to enjoy *eating* food, nor does it encourage early good table manners, and there are the obvious negatives of mess, waste, impracticality and possibly a huge stress factor at mealtimes. Food and eating should be fun, so why not utilise colourful foods and make interesting shapes, patterns and even pictures (see *Party Food* on pages 82–5), and, most obviously, make it taste good!

A baby at this age may also begin to experiment with refusing foods and causing a fuss. This is likely to be a sneaky ploy for attention rather than a true dislike of a taste. If a baby is really determined not to eat the food, just quietly take it away rather than making mealtimes a huge battle. Try the food again another time. Babies may also be easily distracted from the matter in hand – their food. Try eating something at the same time or feeding at the table when others are eating. Babies are excellent mimics and will be more likely to tuck in if they see others doing so.

WHAT TO GIVE

The world of taste continues to open up. Almost all foods can now be eaten by your baby. Fruit and vegetables remain obvious mainstays of a healthy diet for your child. Try varying the texture with grated, roughly cut or diced foods (eg soft fruit or cooked vegetables), in addition to mashed and puréed foods. Berry and citrus fruits can now be given. Different types of cereals, grains and pulses should be offered; potatoes, pasta and bread are all good carbohydrate-packed foods. Experiment with different types of meat (cut any fat off before cooking) and fish (checking carefully for bones), adding oily fish such as mackerel to the repertoire. Now is also a good time to introduce your

WHAT TO GIVE WHEN

baby to flavours such as herbs and garlic which are very beneficial for health and the developing immune system. Only add tiny amounts of these flavourings as these all have very strong tastes. If your baby doesn't like these unusual flavours, leave them for a while, but remember all the individual herbs have very different and individual tastes, so carry on experimenting.

FABULOUS FINGER FOODS

Kids of all ages love finger foods and now is an excellent time to introduce them. They also encourage babies to feed themselves as well as making meals fun. Try the following finger foods:

* Pieces of fruit with pips or stone and skin removed.
* Soft-cooked vegetables in pieces are excellent – steaming is better than boiling to preserve the vitamins. Hard vegetables such as raw carrots are still good for teething.
* Small sandwiches made from soft bread and the range of possible fillings is endless – smooth peanut butter, mashed banana, cottage cheese and grated cucumber, grated cheese and apple, shredded chicken and yoghurt...
* Pasta pieces such as spirals or shells.
* Pieces of bread and toast, pitta bread and chapattis.
* Hard-baked bread or pieces of toast are preferable to sugar-laden rusks for teething.
* Never leave a baby unattended while eating as it is very easy for a small baby to choke. Avoid any foods which are obvious chokers – nuts, fruits with stones and whole grapes. Avoid anything that a baby's gums are going to find hard to break into.

WHAT NOT TO GIVE

The ever-shortening list has dwindled to the obvious trio of sugar, salt and fatty foods. In addition, nuts shouldn't be given

BABY AND TODDLER FOOD

at this age. Cows' milk should also be avoided but now this is not a strict rule.

DRINKS

It is still important to maintain a minimum intake of 1 pint/600ml of formula or breast milk every day (cows' milk is not advised until a baby is a year old, but is fine in small amounts for cooking). This milk is an important source of calcium for developing bones and protein for a growing body. However, up until this time your baby has more than likely been drinking far more than the minimum required one pint of milk. As you increase the amount of solids given this is likely to reduce naturally. If it doesn't, do not worry as long as you have a happy satisfied baby, but if your baby is dissatisfied and unsettled it may be because he or she is drinking too much milk and is not getting the solids needed to prevent hunger pangs. In this case, cut down the milk little by little until the infant is eating more solid food.

Now is also the time to start introducing fruit and vegetable juices. There are many different types and some wonderful combinations can be devised. The ideal is to have your own juice extractor. However, shop-bought juices are still packed full of goodness. Do check it is a pure fruit juice, not some type of 'drink' made with sugar and flavoured water. It is a good idea to dilute the juice, which will also make the carton go much further. The vast weight of evidence points to the wisdom of steering clear of commercial drinks which develop the metaphorical sweet tooth and rot the real ones. If your child is ever given such drinks, do not let them drink them last thing at night or slowly over a prolonged period of time. This is a sure-fire way to encourage dental decay. If you can't give diluted juices, stick to milk or water and offer fresh fruit instead.

WHAT TO GIVE WHEN

Twelve Months and Upwards – Toddlers

At this stage you can start giving your child a smaller portion of what you yourself eat. You may well be surprised by the 'sophisticated' tastes your child likes from a very young age. Make eating a social occasion, as no one really enjoys eating alone. Mealtimes are a central feature of the social fabric of every culture in the world. Once kids launch into terrible toddlerhood they may lose interest in food. After all, it's far more fun to run around and play. But all small children will eat when hungry – toddlers do not starve themselves to death. The other thing to bear in mind is that sometimes tiny stomachs prefer smaller meals more often instead of three big meals a day. In fact, medical opinion seems to be that this could even be a healthier option. Give healthy snacks in between mealtimes such as fruit, raw vegetables, rice cakes or a piece of wholemeal bread. Remember you are developing habits for a lifetime. Toddlers also greatly vary the amount they eat each day: some days they may eat platefuls and other days hardly any food at all. This again is due to only eating when hungry and if you look at the food intake over a few days it will almost certainly be plenty. So unless your child is seriously off their food (which is probably a symptom of being ill) don't panic. For food to capture the interest of a toddler, it only requires a little imagination and patience.

FOOD FUN

- ✱ Let a child 'help' in the kitchen. Small children love to be involved in what you're doing and then they can eat the product of their labours. Plain biscuit dough or pastry is ideal as they can knead it and make it into shapes or use novelty cutters.
- ✱ Arrange food on a plate to form pictures and patterns, using naturally bright-coloured foods for even greater effect. It is no bad thing to be aware of colour contrast

BABY AND TODDLER FOOD

at all times, as brightly coloured foods always look much more appetising.
* Call food or drinks by fun names – look at the commercial foods which sell to children, it's all in the packaging. So 'package' home-made food attractively. Serve Silly Spaghetti, Monster Stew, Dizzy Fizzy water and, of course, Mum's Special Rice.
* Dips with raw vegetable sticks and rice cakes are tremendously healthy and are a different way of eating – novelty value is always a great attention getter.
* Have friends around for tea. If you want your child to eat fish fingers, invite a small friend who loves them and watch your child copy their enthusiasm.
* A change of venue may also work wonders, or even going out for a meal to a café or pizza parlour. In summer, nothing beats a picnic on a nice day – even if it's only in the back garden.
* Food play is useful to encourage interest in mealtimes – make up or read stories involving food, and encourage make-believe play such as food shopping, cooking with toy saucepans, dollies' picnics, and teddies' tea parties.

WHAT TO GIVE

Essentially anything an adult would eat is fine. Make sure it is the right consistency for the child, as a twelve-month-old baby requires soft foods (although it is no longer necessary to purée foods), whereas a two-year-old will eat most textures provided chewy things are cut up. Apart from this, the only thing to remember is to give a balanced, healthy diet – something which should continue for the rest of their lives.

WHAT NOT TO GIVE

Avoid the villainous trio of sugar, salt and fatty foods, and anything a small child might choke on, especially nuts.

WHAT TO GIVE WHEN

FORBIDDEN FRUITS?
As your children grow up and start school you will have less and less control over what they eat. It is important not to make sweet things 'forbidden fruits' as otherwise a child might binge on them when out of the house or view them as an illicit treat. Introduction in moderation is a much better answer. Occasionally have a sweet dessert after lunch or tea instead of the healthier norm of fruit or yoghurts. If your child is given sweets or chocolates, do not take them away, but do insist they are eaten as a dessert after a meal. This is also easier on the teeth and moderates the release of glucose into the system. The other golden rule in relation to sweet things is never to give them as a treat or a bribe. You do not want your child to associate sweets with being good. It is especially important not to use pudding as an incentive to eat a savory course – the first course must be really bad to warrant a bribe! Why not give a piece of exotic fruit, or some dried fruit, or perhaps even a non-food treat such as an outing, special game, comic, balloon or tiny toy. Giving healthy foods as treats or rewards only increases their desirability.

DRINKS
Now that your child is over a year old, it is time to switch to cows' milk. The exception to this is if your child has allergies (see page 88–9). The minimum of a pint a day should still be maintained, but some of this can be substituted with other dairy products such as cheese, yoghurt or fromage frais. Milk shakes are an excellent way for children to consume both milk and vitamin-packed fruit. It is best to give full-fat milk at this stage, or at least semi-skimmed milk. This is because small children probably need more calories from dietary fat than adults. If your child is eating healthily, they should not be overweight. For all other drinks, it is best to stick to diluted fruit and vegetable juices and plain or low-salt fizzy water.

# Table 6
What Weaning When (a)

WHAT TO GIVE		
4-6 months	**6-9 months**	**9-12 months**
Puréed, cooked fruit and vegetables	A wider range of puréed foods of rougher texture, and some larger items to chew on	Almost anything that is wholesome and that the child can swallow, with a wider variety of textures and flavours
Thin porridge made from oat or rice flakes or cornmeal	Puréed, grated or mashed fruit and vegetables	The complete range of fruit and vegetables
	Citrus and soft summer fruits	A variety of breads, grains and pasta
	Tomatoes	Pulses
	Wheat-based foods including cereals and bread	All types of meat and fish
	Well-cooked rice	Well-cooked egg white
	Soft cooked pulses	Dairy products such as yoghurt, fromage frais and cheese
	Purées including chicken, liver and fish	Cow's milk is not advised in large quantities or as a drink, but is acceptable in small quantities in cooking
	Well-cooked egg yolk	Smooth peanut butter and finely ground nuts
	Vitamin drops containing vitamins A, C and D	Vitamin drops containing vitamins A, C and D

Table 6
What Weaning When (b)

WHAT NOT TO GIVE		
4-6 months	**6-9 months**	**9-12 months**
Cow's milk – no milk except breast or formula should be given		
Other dairy products such as yoghurt and cheese		
Wheat and wheat-based products such as wheat cereals		
Tomatoes		
Citrus and soft summer fruits	Cow's milk and other dairy products	
Spices and chillies	Chillies or chilli powder	
Eggs	Egg whites	
Nuts	Nuts	Whole nuts
Salt	Salt	Salt
Sugar	Sugar	Sugar
Fatty foods	Fatty foods	Fatty foods

BABY AND TODDLER FOOD

Table 7
Meal Schedules

	Early morning	Morning (breakfast)	Midday (lunch)	Afternoon (tea)	Evening (bedtime)
1-4 months	Breast/formula milk	Breast/formula milk	Breast/formula milk	Breast/formula milk	Breast/formula milk and a night feed if necessary
4 months	Breast/formula milk	Breast/formula milk	Breast/formula milk and 1-2 tsp purée	Breast/formula milk	Breast/formula milk
Increasing to 5-6 months	Breast/formula milk (if necessary)	Breast/formula milk and a purée	Breast/formula milk and a purée	Breast/formula milk and a purée	Breast/formula milk
6-9 months and 9-12 months	Breast/formula milk (if necessary)	Cereal and breast/formula milk	Protein, vegetables and breast/formula milk	Fruit or vegetables, some toast or bread to chew on and breast/formula milk	Breast/formula milk
1 year upwards	–	Cereal, fruit, cooked breakfast if wished and milk	Protein, vegetables, dairy or fruit pudding and juice and water	Bread (with sandwich filling), fruit and milk or juice and water	Milk

It must be emphasised that this is only a rough guideline. Especially when your child is young, you must follow his/her appetite. As the child becomes older it is easier to follow conventional mealtimes.

4
Recipes

EQUIPMENT
Cooking baby food is not an expensive business and you do not have to buy any extra kitchen equipment. All of these foods can be prepared with a few pots and pans, a fork, a grater and a sieve. However, you may find a blender or food processor particularly useful. I have found a small hand-held blender is ideal, especially when dealing with smaller quantities. The real luxury (for all the family) is a juice extractor, as truly fresh juices have a wonderful taste.

FREEZING
All of these recipes are suitable for freezing, unless otherwise stated. For very young children it is advisable to freeze in tiny quantities (try using an ice-cube tray). As your baby gets older you can freeze in larger portions. Plastic pots or yoghurt cartons (well washed) with a foil cover are ideal. Remember not to keep anything for too long in the freezer; label and date without fail so you know exactly what everything is.

PRODUCE
Fresh foods tend to give the best results, but in many cases frozen or tinned foods can be substituted for convenience. Where herbs are used in the recipes I have generally used fresh; if you want to use dry herbs use one teaspoon measure for each tablespoon. If possible use organic produce as this is both kinder on our bodies and the environment, and often tastes better too. When using an oil always use a vegetable oil such as olive oil or sunflower oil. Choose the unrefined, cold-pressed varieties as they have the highest vitamin content.

BABY AND TODDLER FOOD

TEXTURE

As discussed previously in this *Quick Guide*, you should follow your baby's demands as to the type and amount of food. So, if a recipe is too lumpy for your baby if it is just mashed with a fork, use a blender or sieve. Or try blending the food with a little vegetable purée, or even with some juice or water.

Four–Six Months

All the purées in this section should be made to a smooth consistency and slightly on the runny side. There are many other fruit and vegetables which you could try, but here are some good first-time suggestions. Remember that, at this stage, you should avoid wheat cereals because the early introduction of wheat could trigger a wheat allergy.

CEREALS

Baby rice: This is widely available and should be made up according to the instructions on the packet. Only use those which have no added sugar or salt.

Brown, whole-grain rice: Wash the rice with cold water (the easiest way is to use a sieve under the tap). Simmer in water for about 40 minutes until the grains are tender. Purée using a little baby milk or water to obtain the desired consistency.

Ground rice: Mix 2 tsps ground rice with half a pint of breast or formula milk or water, adding a little at a time. Bring to the boil, stirring continuously. Stir occasionally while it simmers for 5-8 minutes.

Millet: Millet is another gluten-free cereal so is a good wheat substitute. It makes a nice change from rice for very young babies. Mix 2 tsps millet flakes with half a pint of breast or formula milk or water. Bring to the boil, stirring all the time. Stir occasionally while it simmers until it thickens (10-15 minutes).

RECIPES

VEGETABLES

Carrot/broccoli/cauliflower: Peel and slice the carrot, or separate the broccoli or cauliflower into small florets. Simmer in water for about 10 minutes. Purée with a blender or through a sieve, adding a little of the cooking water to obtain a smooth texture.

Courgette: Wash, trim the ends and slice. Simmer for about 5 minutes until tender. (Courgettes steam particularly well, but will need slightly longer – 8–12 minutes.) Purée.

French beans/brussel sprouts: Trim the beans (removing any strings) or sprouts. Simmer for about 8–10 minutes. Purée, using some of the cooking water if necessary.

Leek: Wash well and chop, using only the white part. Simmer for 10–15 minutes. Purée. Leek is a strong taste which a very young baby may not like on its own, but it is excellent combined with potato or parsnip, or some breast or formula milk.

Mushroom: Wash, trim off the stalks, peel and slice. Simmer until tender (8–12 minutes). Purée using some of the cooking water. *Caution:* Mushrooms are fungi and so should be avoided if your baby has a fungal thrush infection.

Peas: Boil the peas until tender – for fresh peas this will be 5–10 minutes; frozen peas will take less time. Purée using some of the cooking water if necessary.

Potato/sweet potato/parsnip/turnip/swede/celeriac: Peel and dice the vegetable. Simmer in water until tender (about 20 minutes). Mash well with a fork, using some of the cooking water to obtain the desired consistency.

Sweet pepper: Remove the stalk, seeds and pith and cut into strips. Simmer for 4–6 minutes. Purée in a blender, or remove the skin and use a fork. Peppers have a distinctive taste and are best when combined with other vegetables.

FRUIT

Apple/pear: Peel and core the fruit (use an eating apple as it will need no added sugar). Chop into pieces, place in a pan and

BABY AND TODDLER FOOD

cover with water. Simmer gently until soft (5–10 minutes). Purée. These purées are excellent for older children and adults. Use as sauces and toppings or stir into plain yoghurt.

Banana: Mash thoroughly 1/4–1/2 of a ripe banana with a fork. It may need a little added cooled, boiled water or breast or formula milk to obtain a smooth purée. *Note:* Banana does not freeze well.

Dried apricots/prunes: Soak the fruit in cold water overnight. Drain and simmer in fresh cold water until soft (10–12 minutes). After removing any stones, push the fruit through a sieve and add sufficient cooking water until it is the right consistency. *Cautions:* Prunes are highly laxative – so use sparingly! All dried fruit, including raisins and sultanas, are common eczema allergens.

Grapes: Halve, peel and remove any seeds to obtain the flesh. Steam for a couple of minutes and purée.

Melon: Cantaloupe melon is especially good as it is packed full of vitamins (notably beta carotene), and has a lovely taste. Cut the melon in half, discard the seeds and scoop out the flesh. Steam for 2–3 minutes and purée.

Peach/apricot/nectarine: Submerge the fruit briefly in boiling water and then in cold water to make peeling easier. Peel the fruit, remove the stone and chop the flesh. Steam for 3–5 minutes and purée.

COMBINATIONS

To create a wider variety of tastes, any of the above purées can be combined with others. If the fruits and/or vegetables you have chosen to combine are cooked in similar ways, you may not have to cook them separately. The following combinations work well:

* broccoli and cauliflower
* carrot and potato
* sweet potato/swede and cauliflower

RECIPES

- tomato and courgette
- mushroom and sweet pepper
- french beans, tomato and pear
- potato and apple
- pear and apricot
- banana and apple
- pear and prune

CREAM OF ...
Another variation of the basic purée which works well is to make a creamy variety. Simply mix the purée with some baby rice or some breast or formula milk. Your baby may prefer the creamier taste.

Six–nine Months

Any of the purées in the previous section can be used, made to a thicker consistency. Reduce the amount of any added water, and cut down the cooking time slightly to help preserve vitamins. The purées below are good ones to add to the repertoire. Melons, grapes and pears, puréed previously, can now be eaten raw – mash the ripe flesh with a fork. In fact, any fruits which are soft enough should now be eaten uncooked. For many of the harder fruits, such as apple, grating does the trick to make it edible for tiny mouths. Raw is great for instant meals and ensuring that all the goodness is preserved. It is often good to mix the sweeter fruits with other savory tastes. Again, the combinations are limitless, so use your imagination.

CEREALS
Weetabix: Soak half a Weetabix in breast or formula milk, or diluted apple juice for a few minutes. Purée once soft. As your baby gets better at chewing, the soaked Weetabix will only need

BABY AND TODDLER FOOD

mashing. Weetabix makes an excellent combination with grated or puréed apple.

Oat porridge: Bring 3–4 tbsps of formula or breast milk to the boil. Add about 1/2 tbsp of rolled porridge oats. Stir as it simmers for 1–1 1/2 minutes. Leave to stand for a couple of minutes. Add more milk or water if it is too thick.

Barley and vegetable soup: A hearty, nourishing soup that satisfies the hungriest of stomachs. The amount above makes two adult portions, so would make more than enough for mother and baby (for adults it tastes great with added ginger and black pepper). This recipe works particularly well with root vegetables, such as carrot, parsnip and swede.

1 tbsp cold-pressed olive oil
1 onion, peeled and chopped
225g (8oz) any colourful vegetable, chopped, diced or shredded
40g (1 1/2oz) pot barley
600ml (1 pint) vegetable stock (no salt added)

Heat the oil and lightly sauté the onions and the other vegetable of your choice. Stir in the pot barley and stock. Cover and simmer over a low heat for 2 hours or until the barley is soft. Purée.

Oat and vegetable medley:

3 tbsps porridge oats
200g (7oz) mixture of vegetables (such as potato, parsnip, leek, onion, celery, carrot, broccoli), chopped as appropriate
Water or chicken stock (see below) as required

This is a variation on the barley and vegetable soup. Place the oats and vegetables in a saucepan. Cover with water or chicken stock and simmer for 20 minutes. Purée.

CHICKEN

Chicken purée: Cover a chicken breast with water and simmer for 20 minutes. Purée using some of the cooking water to obtain the right consistency. Alternatively, a purée can be made using chopped leftover roast chicken and water. This purée tastes great mixed with a little spinach and apple.

Chicken stock: Home-made chicken stock has many uses and is especially good for soups and casseroles. It also makes full use of the chicken carcass after the meat has been eaten. Make a batch and freeze in portions for easy use.

Chicken bones and giblets
Any leftover chicken meat, chopped (optional)
2 medium onions, peeled and roughly chopped
1 parsnip, chopped
2–3 carrots, peeled and chopped
2 leeks, chopped
1 celery stalk, chopped
1 tbsp chopped fresh parsley

Place all the ingredients in a large saucepan. Cover with plenty of water. Simmer for 2½–3 hours adding more water if necessary. Leave to cool and skim off the fat from the surface. Strain the mixture and keep the stock in the fridge. Home-made stock is especially useful as it does not contain salt or additives such as monosodium glutamate which are added to most commercial stock cubes.

Chicken casserole:

1 chicken breast, chopped
1 medium potato, scrubbed and chopped
1 small parsnip, peeled and chopped
1 small carrot, peeled and chopped
½ celery stalk, chopped
250ml (8fl oz) chicken stock (see above), or water

Place all the ingredients in a saucepan with a lid. Simmer for about 30 minutes. Purée all of the meat and vegetables together.

BABY AND TODDLER FOOD

Chicken with lentils and apple:
50g (2oz) cooked chicken, chopped
50g (2oz) lentils, cooked (see page 54)
1 small eating apple, peeled, cored and grated
2 tbsps apple juice or water (if required)

Purée all the ingredients together using as much of the juice as is necessary to make it a good texture.

LIVER

Liver is an excellent source of iron. However if your baby still prefers bland tastes, it is probably best to introduce liver once he or she is around twelve months' old.

Liver, leek and potato:
50g (2oz) calves liver
1 medium potato, scrubbed and finely chopped
2 leeks (white part only), chopped
120ml (4fl oz) chicken stock (see page 51)

Place all the ingredients in a saucepan and cover. Simmer gently for 10 minutes. Purée. Serve with rice or potato.

FISH

White fish: For this recipe, defrosted frozen fish can be used, which means it is an easy dish for you to keep all the ingredients to hand. Place a fillet or piece of bone-free white fish (eg cod, haddock, coley, plaice or whiting) on an oiled piece of aluminium foil, in an oven-proof dish. Pour about 2 tbsps of breast or formula milk or water over the fish. A dash of lemon juice can be added. Bring the sides of the foil up and fold together so the fish is encased. Bake in a preheated oven at 180°C (gas mark 4, 350°F) for about 20 minutes. Purée. Serve with puréed vegetables.

RECIPES

Cod in tomato:
1 fillet of cod
2 tomatoes, skinned, seeded and chopped
80ml (3fl oz) water
dash of lemon juice

Place the cod into an oven-proof dish. Cover with the tomatoes, lemon juice and water. Cover and bake in a preheated oven at 180°C (gas mark 4, 350°F) for 20 minutes. Purée the fish in the liquid it is cooked in. Serve with potato.

Cod with rice and spinach:
1 fillet of cod
100g (4oz) spinach, stalks removed
80ml (3fl oz) water
50g (2oz) brown rice, well cooked

Bake the cod and spinach in the water in a preheated oven at 180°C (gas mark 4, 350°F) for 20 minutes. Purée the fish and spinach with the rice.

Plaice with cauliflower and mushroom:
1 fillet of plaice
Few cauliflower florets, chopped
Few mushrooms, chopped
80ml (3fl oz) water

Put all the ingredients together in an oven-proof dish and cover. Bake in a preheated oven at 180°C (gas mark 4, 350°F) for 20 minutes. Purée with the liquid it is cooked in.

Tuna: Another convenient food to keep to hand. Use tinned tuna in vegetable oil. Drain well and mash with some water or a vegetable purée. Tuna combines excellently with tomato, cauliflower or apple.

BABY AND TODDLER FOOD

PULSES

Pulses are an excellent source of protein and important minerals. They make ideal baby foods, being nutritious and easy to purée. They also have a good texture which many babies find very palatable. Soak in cold water and cook according to the following table. *Caution:* All pulses *must* be boiled rapidly for at least 20 minutes before simmering. This is to remove toxic substances naturally present. Always drain off the soaking water and cook in fresh water. These purées are best mixed with other vegetables initially and they taste great combined with swede, leek or potato. All cooked pulses freeze well. Tinned pulses are also a useful stand-by.

Table 8
Cooking Pulses

	SOAKING	COOKING
Aduki beans	no need	35–40 minutes
Black-eyed beans	no need	40–50 minutes
Borlotti beans	overnight	60–70 minutes
Butter beans	overnight	1–1^1/$_2$ hours
Chick peas	overnight	2–3 hours
Dried peas	overnight	1^1/$_2$–2 hours
Flageolet beans	overnight	1 hour
Haricot beans	overnight	50–60 minutes
Lentils	no need	30–40 minutes
Red kidney beans	overnight	1^1/$_2$–2 hours
Mung beans	no need	40–50 minutes
Pinto beans	overnight	1^1/$_2$–2 hours
Soya beans	overnight	3^1/$_2$–4 hours

RECIPES

VEGETABLES

Spinach: Wash the leaves and remove the stalks. Simmer for 5–8 minutes until tender. Purée.

Tomato: Submerge the tomatoes briefly in boiling water and then in cold water. Peel, remove the seeds and chop the flesh into a saucepan. Heat gently for a couple of minutes before puréeing. Tinned tomatoes work well in most recipes.

FRUIT

Berries (eg blackberries, raspberries and strawberries): Wash, remove any stalks and discard any blemished fruit. Steam for 3–5 minutes, or boil briefly if necessary to soften. Purée. Such fruits can often have a tart taste and may be more palatable combined with another fruit such as eating apples. Berries contain many tiny seeds which are designed to be indigestible, passing through the body, so these will not affect your baby. It is only worth removing the seeds by sieving if your baby objects to them!

Cherries: Obtain the flesh by halving, peeling and removing the stones. Mash with a fork.

Citrus fruits (eg oranges, grapefruits, mandarins): Peel, remove pith and any pips. Divide into segments and purée in a blender. If too tart, mix with other sweeter fruits. Citrus fruits combine very well with banana.

Dried dates: Chop and remove any stones. Simmer until tender (about 5–10 minutes). Purée. Dates are very sweet and have a high fructose content so are better mixed with other foods. This purée is also very useful as a natural sweetener for foodstuffs and puddings for all the family.

Kiwi: Cut in half, scoop out the flesh and purée. This may then need to be pushed through a fine sieve to remove the seeds. Older children can eat kiwis like a boiled egg. Simply slice the top off and scoop out the delicious insides with a teaspoon.

Mango/avocado/plums: Cut a ripe fruit in half (avocados are

BABY AND TODDLER FOOD

ripe when the skins are just beginning to turn black) and ease it away from the stone. Scoop the flesh out of the skin and mash thoroughly with a fork. None of these fruits freeze well. Some babies may find avocado too rich to digest, so use sparingly in the early stages.

Papaya: Cut the fruit in half, remove the seeds and scoop out the flesh. Mash well with a fork. *Note:* Papaya does not freeze well.

Nine–Twelve Months

MEAT

Chicken and leek with baked potato: For baby, just serve the soft mixture. But for the rest of the family, spoon the mixture on to the potato, obtaining the full goodness of their fibre and vitamin C.

4 baking potatoes
2 leeks, sliced
2–3 slices cooked chicken, chopped
few black olives, finely chopped (optional)
black pepper to season
175g (6oz) low-fat fromage frais
1 tbsp fresh parsley, chopped

Bake the potatoes for 1¼ hours at 190°C (gas mark 5, 375°F). Meanwhile, steam the leeks until soft. Mix in the ham and olives and warm through. Cut the baked potatoes in half lengthways and scoop out the flesh. Mix the potato flesh with the chicken, leeks and fromage frais. Season with black pepper. Return the mixture to the potato skins and sprinkle with the parsley.

Marvellous mince: If you have troublesome toddlers who don't eat their veggies, mince is a master of disguise, full of goodness. Boost its nutritional content with a healthy dose of carrots and finely chopped vegetables in a rich tomato sauce.

RECIPES

> 225g (8oz) lean mince beef or lamb
> 1 onion, peeled and chopped
> 1 green pepper, seeded and chopped
> 50g (2oz) mushrooms, chopped
> 2 carrots, thinly sliced
> 450g (14oz) tin chopped tomatoes
> 1 tbsp tomato purée (see page 55)
> 1 tbsp fresh oregano, chopped or (1 tsp dried mixed herbs)
> 1 clove of garlic, crushed (optional)
> 1 tbsp olive oil
> black pepper to season

Gently fry the onion in the olive oil until translucent. Add the mince and garlic. Fry the meat until cooked through. Drain the fatty juices away before transferring to a large saucepan. Add the rest of the ingredients and simmer for 20–30 minutes, stirring occasionally. Serve with small pieces of pasta, rice or mashed potatoes.

Chicken and orange with rice: This simple recipe can be used to great effect with leftover chicken from a roast and only takes a minute to throw together.

> 400g (14oz) cooked brown rice
> 2 pieces cooked chicken, chopped
> 2 oranges, peeled and chopped
> 1 tbsp fresh parsley, chopped
> black pepper to season

Mix all the ingredients together. Lovely cold, this can also be warmed through in the microwave. If it is a little dry add a tablespoon of orange juice. The baby's portion needs a quick whizz in a blender.

FISH

Granny's fish pie: This simple dish is a delicious mixture of fish. Use any of the white fishes, salmon, tuna and some tinned shrimps or crab for an exotic touch.

BABY AND TODDLER FOOD

350g (12oz) fish
1 onion, peeled and chopped
1/2 tbsp olive oil
1 egg, hardboiled, chopped
1/4 pint semi-skimmed milk
juice of 1 lemon
1 tbsp fresh parsley, chopped
1 tbsp fresh dill, chopped
750g (11/2lb) potatoes
black pepper to season
handful of grated cheddar cheese (optional)

Fry the onion in the olive oil until translucent. Place the fish with the milk, egg, onion, lemon juice and chopped herbs in an oven-proof dish. Cover and bake for 20 minutes at 180°C (gas mark 4, 350°F). Meanwhile, boil the potatoes until soft and mash with some black pepper. Cover the fish with the mashed potato. For the older folks it is lovely to sprinkle some grated cheese on the top and brown under a hot grill. Serve with a green vegetable such as broccoli or puréed carrot.

Cod with apple:

4 pieces of cod
juice of 1 lemon
2 eating apples, cored, peeled and sliced

Place the cod on a greased piece of foil. Cover with the apple slices and lemon juice. Sprinkle with the grated nutmeg. Pull the sides of the foil together over the top to make a parcel. Bake in the oven for 20 minutes at 180°C (gas mark 4, 350°F). Serve with mixed brown rices and a puréed vegetable for a gourmet meal.

Crumbed plaice: This is the easy way to make crumbed fish and is very healthy as it does not need any frying.

4 fillets of plaice
juice of 1 lemon

75g (3oz) wholemeal breadcrumbs
25g (1oz) ground almonds
40g (1½oz) hard cheese, grated
1 tbsp olive oil

Place the fish and lemon juice in a greased oven-proof dish. Toss the breadcrumbs, almonds and cheese in the olive oil. Cover the fish with the topping and season with black pepper. Place under a hot grill until the fish is cooked and the crumb topping is starting to brown (about 10 minutes).

PULSES

Hummus: This is also a delicious filling for sandwiches or baked potatoes, or is very tasty on rye crackers or rice cakes. I keep a tub in the fridge for the entire family.

50g (2oz) cooked chick peas
juice of 1 lemon
2 cloves of garlic, peeled and crushed
1 tbsp cold-pressed olive oil
1 tbsp tahini (smooth sesame-seed paste)
50ml (2fl oz) water (optional)
fresh parsley to garnish

If using a food processor, place all the ingredients in a bowl and blend until smooth. Alternatively, place all the ingredients into a large mixing bowl and pound with a potato masher, if necessary adding a little water to make the mixture smooth. Add to vegetable purées or serve on its own on triangles of wholemeal bread.

Baked beans: All kids love baked beans. These are easy to cook and much tastier than the tinned varieties.

1 tbsp olive oil
1 onion, peeled and finely chopped
400g (14oz) tinned tomatoes
1 tbsp tomato purée (see page 55)

BABY AND TODDLER FOOD

2 tsps fresh basil, chopped
250g (9oz) dried haricot beans (see page 54) or 800g (2 x 14oz) tinned haricot beans

Heat the olive oil and fry the onion until transparent. Add the tomatoes, tomato purée and basil and stir. Add the beans and cook for several minutes until heated through.

Pinto bean casserole:

225g (8oz) pinto beans, cooked (see page 56)
1 onion, peeled and chopped
1 large parsnip, peeled and chopped
2 carrots, peeled and sliced
1 leek, trimmed and sliced
1 tbsp sesame seeds
1/2 tin (3oz) chopped tomatoes in tomato juice
1/2 tbsp tomato purée (see page 57)
300ml (1/2 pint) vegetable stock
1 tbsp olive oil
1 tbsp fresh mixed herbs, chopped
black pepper to season

Fry the onion in the oil until translucent in a large saucepan. Then add the parsnip, carrots and leek and cook for a few minutes more. Add all the remaining ingredients and bring to the boil. Simmer for 20–30 minutes. Serve with wholemeal bread or rice.

PASTA

Tuna and sweetcorn: An eternal favourite! This dish also freezes well without the yoghurt, which can be added when reheating.

225g (8oz) pasta shapes, eg macaroni or spirals
1 tin (185g) tuna in vegetable oil
1 tin (198g) sweetcorn
200g (7oz) Greek-style yoghurt

50g (2oz) hard cheese, grated
black pepper to season
1 tbsp fresh dill, chopped (optional)

Cook the pasta in boiling water until still slightly firm. Drain. Drain the tuna and sweetcorn and add with the rest of the ingredients to the pasta. Stir well and heat through before serving.

Chicken and courgette shells:
225g (8oz) pasta shells
2 pieces of cooked chicken, chopped
½ large onion, peeled and chopped
2 large courgettes, sliced
1 carton passata (sieved tomatoes)
1 tbsp fresh marjoram, chopped
1 clove of garlic, crushed
½ tbsp olive oil

Fry the onion in the olive oil until translucent. Add the courgettes and sauté for a couple of minutes. Then add the passata, chicken, garlic and marjoram. Cover and leave to simmer for 10 minutes. Meanwhile, cook the pasta in boiling water until still slightly firm. Drain the pasta and serve with the sauce. Younger babies' portions may need to be chopped smaller in the blender.

VEGETABLES

Puréed carrots with basil: This delicious vegetable dish can be served with fish, meat or casserole dishes. It is worth using extra-virgin olive oil as the flavour comes across very well. Any leftover purée can be added to soups, stocks or risotto dishes. Wonderful for adding to a meal of any age group – including adults!

450g (1lb) carrots, scrubbed and sliced
2 tsps extra-virgin olive oil
2 tbsps freshly squeezed orange juice
1 tbsp fresh basil, chopped

BABY AND TODDLER FOOD

Cook the carrots by placing in boiling water. Reserve the cooking liquid for future use as a vegetable stock or soup base. Place the cooked carrots in a food processor or liquidiser. Purée until smooth. Add the olive oil, orange juice and chopped basil. Purée again and serve immediately while still hot.

Watercress and spinach rice:

350g (12oz) cooked brown rice
100g (4oz) fresh spinach
1 tsp nut butter (see pages 69–70)
1/2 tbsp olive oil
1 egg, beaten

Remove tough stems from the watercress and spinach. Blend the nut butter and oil over a gentle heat. Add the leaves and cook until wilted. Mix in the cooked rice, turn up the heat and warm through. Pour the egg over the rice and carry on cooking for a few minutes, stirring until the egg is cooked through. Chop leaves into small pieces before serving.

Tomato and vegetable soup: This nourishing soup is quick and easy to make. An excellent nutritional booster for children.

125g (4oz) celery, chopped with its leaves
125g (4oz) carrot, grated
50g (2oz) raw spinach, finely chopped
1 litre (1 3/4 pints) water
125ml (4fl oz) tomato juice
1 tsp honey
black pepper to season
1 tbsp chopped fresh chives (optional)

Boil the water in a pan and add the chopped vegetables. Cover, turn down the heat and simmer for 20–30 minutes. Add the tomato juice and seasonings of honey and pepper. Pour into a blender and liquidise until smooth. Serve with a sprinkling of chopped chives.

RECIPES

FRUIT AND YOGHURT
Older babies enjoy dairy products such as yoghurt. Try giving your baby plain yoghurt to begin with (this can be sweetened with a few drops of natural maple syrup). Later, this can be mixed with many different fruit purées.

Twelve Months and Upwards – Toddlers

CEREALS
Bircher muesli: This recipe is based on the original muesli invented by Dr Bircher-Benner for patients at his famous natural health clinic in Switzerland. Older children and adults may enjoy it with a sprinkling of finely chopped hazelnuts.

4 tbsps rolled oats
2 tbsps low-fat yoghurt
6 tbsps cold water
1/2 tsp grated lemon rind
225g (8oz) freshly grated apple

Place the oats, yoghurt, water and lemon rind into a large bowl and stir. Leave in the fridge overnight. Add the fruit and serve.

Apricot and orange muesli:

4 tbsps rolled oats
275g (10oz) dried apricots, chopped
1/2 tsp grated orange rind
150ml (5fl oz) orange juice
milk or yoghurt as required

Soak the oats, apricots, orange juice and rind overnight in the fridge. Add milk or yoghurt as required and serve. For older children, a sprinkling of chopped nuts adds the finishing touch.

Commercial breakfast cereals: Now that your child is a year old and can drink cow's milk, breakfast cereals are an excellent

Table 9
Breakfast Cereals

Cereal	Total fats (g)	Total sugars (g)	Calories (kcal)
All Bran	2.5	19.0	261
Bran Flakes	1.6	18.7	318
Coco Pops	0.9	38.2	384
Corn Flakes	0.5	8.2	360
Crunchy Nut Corn Flakes	3.8	36.3	398
Frosties	0.4	41.9	377
Muesli *(average)*	5.2	26.2	363
Muesli *(no added sugar)*	7.4	15.7	366
Oat Bran Flakes	2.4	16.8	357
Porridge *(made with water)*	1.0	almost nil	49
Porridge *(made with full-fat milk)*	4.7	4.7	116
Puffed Wheat	1.0	0.3	321
Ready Brek (plain)	6.6	1.7	373
Rice Krispies	0.8	10.6	369
Ricicles	0.5	41.9	381
Shredded Wheat	2.2	0.8	325
Shreddies	1.1	10.2	331
Smacks	1.5	50.0	386
Special K	0.9	17.2	377
Start	1.4	29.1	355
Sugar Puffs	0.6	56.5	324
Weetabix	2.0	5.2	352
Weetos	1.9	33.2	372

(measurements per 100g)

and easy start to the day. Good varieties include Weetabix, Ready Brek (plain), Rice Krispies, Puffed Wheat, Shredded Wheat and good old-fashioned porridge oats. But, be aware that many commercial cereals are packed full of fat and sugar – some even contain more sugar than a Mars bar! Just take a glance at Table 9.

MEAT

Beautiful bangers: These are simple to make and you have the reassurance that these delicious home-made sausages really are packed full of meat.

750g (1½lb) pork, minced
1 large onion, peeled and roughly chopped
1 tsp French mustard
2 large free-range eggs
1 tbsp fresh sage, chopped (optional)
25g (1oz) buckwheat flour or barley flour

Mix all the ingredients apart from the flour in a food processor until the mixture resembles sausage meat (this may take a few minutes). Flour your hands and roll the mixture into sausage shapes or small patties. Cook under a preheated grill, turning several times.

Beef and mushroom casserole: For adults this recipe also tastes great with red wine. So half-way through the cooking time take out baby's portion and add a generous splash to the rest!

350g (12oz) lean stewing beef, trimmed and cut into small pieces
1 large onion, peeled and sliced
1 tbsp olive oil
225g (8oz) potatoes, cut into chunks
600ml (1 pint) vegetable stock
100g (4oz) button mushrooms, quartered
1 tbsp tomato purée (see page 55)
1 clove of garlic, crushed
1 tbsp fresh rosemary, chopped

BABY AND TODDLER FOOD

Fry the onion in the oil until translucent. Add the stewing beef and fry until the outsides are evenly browned. Place all the ingredients in a casserole dish, cover and cook at 180°C (gas mark 4, 350°F) for 1½–2 hours. The casserole may need some extra liquid adding half way through the cooking time. Serve with a green vegetable and hunks of wholemeal bread.

Chicken and broccoli bake:
   4 pieces of chicken, chopped
   broccoli, separated into florets
   25g (1oz) butter
   25g (1oz) wholemeal flour
   ½ pint skimmed or semi-skimmed milk
   1 tbsp fresh parsley, chopped
   black pepper to season
   200g (8oz) wholemeal breadcrumbs
   25g (1oz) ground almonds
   50g (2oz) hard cheese, grated
   1½ tbsps olive oil

Chop the chicken into bite-sized pieces. Place the chicken and broccoli in an oven-proof dish. Melt the margarine, blend in the flour. Gradually add the milk, stirring continuously. Bring to the boil and simmer for a couple of minutes. Stir in the herbs and pour over the chicken and broccoli. Season with black pepper. Cover and bake in a preheated oven for 30–35 minutes at 180°C (gas mark 4, 350°F). Meanwhile, toss the breadcrumbs, ground almonds and cheese in the olive oil. Ten minutes before the chicken is cooked, remove the cover and sprinkle on the crumb topping. Replace in the oven for the remaining cooking time.

Chicken and mango salad: This is a delicious dish for a summer lunch or light supper. In the unlikely event of any being left over, use to stuff pitta bread or serve warm on a bed of brown rice.

6 pieces of cooked chicken
1 medium onion, peeled and roughly chopped
1 ripe mango
small bunch seedless grapes

For the dressing:
85ml (3fl oz) sunflower or safflower oil
1 tbsp white wine vinegar or cider vinegar
1 tsp honey
1 tbsp plain, low-fat, live yoghurt

Cut the chicken into bite-sized pieces. Peel the mango and cut into cubes roughly the same size as the chicken pieces. Wash the grapes and remove the stalks. Place the chicken pieces into a large mixing bowl, add the mango and grapes and mix together. Make the dressing by whisking all the ingredients together in a jug or bowl. Alternatively, put all the ingredients into a screw-top jar and shake well to mix. Pour the dressing over the chicken salad and toss with a spoon. Serve on wholemeal pasta cooked in the chicken stock or new potatoes still in their skins.

FISH

Fishy soup: This hearty Spanish soup is both nutritious and filling. It is also a good way of using up leftover rice. Alternatively, use Whole Earth's precooked tinned brown rice which has a good flavour and is a great time saver.

1kg (2lb) firm-fleshed fish, eg cod, hoki or hake
1 litre (1³/₄ pints) water
2 tbsps olive oil
3 cloves of garlic, crushed
1 medium onion, chopped
8 large tomatoes, chopped
1 red pepper, deseeded and chopped
¹/₂kg (1lb) new potatoes, scrubbed
300g (11oz) cooked brown rice
50g (2oz) fresh parsley, finely chopped

BABY AND TODDLER FOOD

Briefly fry the fish in 1 tablespoon of the olive oil. Flake into large chunks and remove any bones. Place the bones in a saucepan with the water, remaining olive oil, garlic, onion, tomatoes and seasoning. Bring to the boil, cover and simmer for 30–40 minutes. Strain the liquid through a sieve and add the new potatoes. Simmer gently for 20 minutes or until the potatoes have softened. Add the cooked brown rice and adjust the seasoning. Just before serving, stir in the pieces of fish and sprinkle with freshly chopped parsley.

Fish cakes: This recipe works well with cod, coley and hoki (an inexpensive fish from New Zealand available at most supermarkets), or try it with salmon for the grown-ups!

550g (1¼lb) potatoes, scrubbed
2 tbsps cold-pressed olive oil
1 large onion, peeled and finely chopped
450g (1lb) fresh (or frozen and defrosted) fish fillets
1 tbsp fresh thyme, chopped
juice of ½ lemon
1 egg, lightly beaten
4-6 tbsps sesame seeds for coating

Preheat the oven to 190°C (gas mark 5, 375°F). Boil the potatoes until cooked, drain and mash them with 1 tablespoon of the olive oil. Heat the other tablespoon of olive oil and fry the onion and fish until the fish is white and the onion is transparent. Mix the fish and onion with the mashed potato and add the thyme, lemon juice and egg, stirring well. Mould the mixture into 12 small round, flat fish cakes. Coat with the sesame seeds. Bake for 15–20 minutes until cooked through.

Fast fish risotto: This risotto is a good way to use up precooked rice. For even more convenience tinned fish such as tuna or salmon may be substituted for the fresh oily fish. Babies are surprisingly adventurous in their tastes and often like the unusual flavour of mackerel or herring. Mix with vegetable purées to make it suitable for the nine- to twelve-month age group.

100g (4oz) fresh oily fish (eg mackerel or herring)
1 onion, peeled and finely chopped
1 tbsp olive oil
6 heaped tbsps cooked brown rice
150g (5oz) frozen peas
1 tbsp fresh parsley, chopped

Cook the fish under a hot grill for about 5 minutes, turning it once. Allow to cool slightly, then flake the fish flesh into large pieces. Heat the oil in a large frying pan and lightly fry the onion. Add the fish, the rice and peas. Stir continuously to prevent the mixture sticking to the sides of the saucepan while heating through for about 3 minutes to cook the peas. Sprinkle with the parsley before serving.

PULSES AND NUTS

Bean and flour patties: The gram flour used in this recipe comes from ground chick peas and gives the patties a distinctive flavour and golden colour. They are very popular with children of all ages.

100g (4oz) gram flour
300ml (1/2 pint) skimmed, semi-skimmed or soya milk
1 tbsp olive oil
175g (6oz) cooked aduki beans (see page 54)
1 tbsp mixed fresh oregano and thyme, chopped

Sieve the flour into a basin and stir in the milk to make a light batter. Heat the oil in a frying pan and add spoonfuls of the batter. Sprinkle 2 tsps aduki beans on each pattie before turning to fry on the other side. Remove from the pan and keep the patties warm while you cook the remaining batter.

Nut butter: Nut butter with chopped celery makes an unusual and tasty filling for sandwiches and baked potatoes in their jackets. But nut butter is far more versatile than just a spread –

BABY AND TODDLER FOOD

try dabbing a little over cooked carrots, or adding 1/2 teaspoon to a salad dressing for extra flavour. Cashew nuts have the highest fat content, so use sparingly. Hazelnuts are the lowest in fat, while almonds are the richest in vitamin E.

450g (1lb) mixture of almonds, brazil nuts, walnuts, hazelnuts or peanuts

4 tbsps apple juice

Roast the nuts in a medium oven for 10–15 minutes, stirring occasionally. Grind to a fine paste in a coffee mill or food processor with a sharp blade. Stir in just enough apple juice to make a thick purée. Store in screw-top jars. If the natural oil in the nuts separates, simply stir it back in. You can also make this recipe using seeds. For seeds such as sesame or sunflower, dry roast in a pan over a low heat until the seeds crush easily when rubbed. Then proceed as before.

Soya bean bake:

8 tbsps soya beans, canned or precooked (see page 54)
1 egg yolk
1/2 onion, peeled and chopped
1/2 tbsp olive oil
2oz (50g) mushrooms, diced
1 eating apple, peeled, cored and chopped
1 tbsp fresh marjoram, chopped
2 tbsps semi-skimmed milk
2 tbsps ground almonds

Fry the onion in olive oil until translucent, then add the mushrooms and slice for another couple of minutes. Mix in the rest of the ingredients, apart from the ground almonds. Tip the mixture into a greased casserole dish. Sprinkle with the ground almonds. Cover and bake for 30-35 minutes at 180°C (gas mark 4, 350°F). If the bake is not soft enough for baby, moisten with a tablespoon of apple juice or passata (sieved tomatoes).

RECIPES

Pasta

Pasta pomodoro: This rich tomato sauce can be used for pasta, rice or even leftover fish. I always make twice the quantity as it keeps for up to a week in the fridge or for up to 3 months in the freezer. Passata (sieved tomatoes) is a good substitute for whole tomatoes and works well in this recipe. Cartons or jars of passata can be found in most supermarkets.

120ml (4fl oz) olive oil
300g (10oz) onion, finely chopped
100g (4oz) carrot, chopped
4 cloves of garlic, crushed
1kg (2¼lb) tomatoes, chopped or 1 litre (1¾ pint) passata
1 tbsp fresh basil, chopped
1 tbsp fresh oregano, chopped
100g (4oz) dried wholemeal pasta per person
parmesan cheese, grated (optional)

Heat the oil in a large saucepan or deep-sided frying pan. Add the onions, carrot and garlic. Stir frequently until the vegetables have softened. Add the chopped tomatoes or passata, cover the pan and simmer over a low heat for 20 minutes. Stir in the herbs, partially cover and simmer for a further 10 minutes.

Cook the pasta until still slightly firm, drain and serve immediately with a helping of the pomodoro sauce. Sprinkle with freshly grated parmesan cheese.

Popeye pie: This tasty pasta pie freezes well, so make an extra one for the freezer. If you can't find fresh spinach, use a block of frozen spinach which has just as many vitamins and also cuts down the preparation time.

300g (11oz) dried wholewheat macaroni
450g (1lb) fresh spinach or 225g (8oz) frozen spinach, thawed
50ml (2fl oz) skimmed milk
1 medium onion, chopped
3 cloves of garlic, crushed and chopped

BABY AND TODDLER FOOD

small piece root ginger, grated
100g (4oz) wholewheat breadcrumbs
50g (2oz) parmesan cheese, grated
25g (1oz) sesame seeds

Preheat the oven to 190°C (gas mark 5, 375°F). Cook the macaroni according to the instructions on the packet. Rinse in cold water to stop the cooking process and drain. If using fresh spinach, wash and chop into small pieces. Cook by plunging into boiling water for 2–3 minutes. Place the spinach in a large mixing bowl. Add the milk, onion, garlic and grated ginger root to season. Stir in the cooked macaroni and transfer to a baking dish. Mix together the breadcrumbs, parmesan cheese and sesame seeds. Sprinkle liberally over the macaroni mixture. Bake in the preheated oven for 20–25 minutes or until the breadcrumb topping is crisp and golden.

'Spag bol': Children love to eat long strings of spaghetti and seem to manage to get most of it into their mouths one way or another.

300–400g (12oz) dried spaghetti
1 portion of Marvellous Mince (see pages 56–7)
parmesan cheese, grated (optional)

Cook the pasta until still slightly firm. Drain and roughly chop into shorter strands. Serve with the mince and a generous sprinkling of grated parmesan cheese.

Pasta parcels: Although these are very fiddly to make, many supermarkets and shops stock excellent fresh pasta 'parcels'. (Remember to read the labels before you buy.) These are stuffed with a variety of fillings, including cheese, spinach or meat. They are excellent served with a fresh vegetable such as broccoli or courgettes and are useful convenience foods.

VEGETABLES

Cauliflower cheese: This is popular with all the family. Any hard cheese can be used so experiment with different tastes such as Gruyère and goat's cheese. For a baby's portion, just mash the cauliflower and sauce together with a fork.

350g (12oz) cauliflower
25g (1oz) butter
25g (1oz) wholemeal flour
300ml (1/2 pint) skimmed or semi-skimmed milk
100g (4oz) cheese, grated
1 tbsp fresh parsley, chopped

Separate the cauliflower into small florets and cook until tender. When cooked, place in dish. Meanwhile, melt the butter over a low heat, blend in the flour and stir for a couple of minutes over the heat. Gradually add the milk, stirring continuously. Bring almost to the boil and simmer for a couple of minutes. Stir in the cheese and pour over the cauliflower. Sprinkle on the parsley and serve.

Red pepper rafts: A no-fuss teatime dish that looks impressive but takes no time to put together. Serve on a colourful sea of shredded spring greens, spinach or savoy cabbage.

4 large red peppers
1 medium onion, finely chopped
50ml (2fl oz) olive oil
100g (4oz) grated carrot
200g (7oz) long-grain brown rice
600ml (1 pint) vegetable or chicken stock
275g (10oz) packet of frozen peas
75g (3oz) seedless raisins
1/2 tsp dried thyme
1 tbsp fresh parsley, chopped

Preheat the oven to 190°C (gas mark 5, 375°F). In a large pan lightly fry the onion in the olive oil, add the carrot and rice, stir well. Pour in the stock, add the peas, raisins, thyme, and salt and pepper to season. Prepare the peppers by removing their stalks (push the stalks down into the pepper, twist and remove). Rinse

BABY AND TODDLER FOOD

the seeds out from inside each one. Slice each pepper cleanly in half. Place on a non-stick baking sheet and bake for 15–20 minutes. Remove from the oven and stuff with the rice mixture. Sprinkle with the chopped parsley. Serve hot.

Carrot soup: This soup is an amazingly good source of beta carotene, but above all, it tastes delicious!

8 large carrots, scrubbed and sliced
600ml (1 pint) water
600ml (1 pint) vegetable stock (home made or a low-salt cube)
1 tbsp chopped fresh coriander or parsley
small carton plain, low-fat yoghurt (140g)
chopped chives to garnish

Cook the carrots in the water with the vegetable stock. Add the chopped herbs and seasonings. Purée in a blender or food processor until smooth. Serve in small bowls with a swirl of plain yoghurt and a sprinkling of chopped chives to garnish.

Sweet potato and mushroom risotto: A gourmet meal for all the family. Experiment with using a mixture of rices (eg brown basmati and brown Italian rice) for added variety.

100g (4oz) brown rice, well rinsed
475ml (16fl oz) water
1 large onion, peeled and finely chopped
100g (4oz) sweet potato, scrubbed and diced
2 tsps olive oil
100g (4oz) mushrooms, finely chopped
2 tbsps fresh parsley, chopped (keep a few sprigs for a garnish)
juice of ½ lemon

Gently heat a heavy-based saucepan on top of the stove, add the rice and stir with a wooden spatula for 1 minute until lightly toasted. Add the water and onion. Bring to the boil, cover and simmer for 20 minutes. Add the sweet potato and simmer for another 10-15 minutes until the rice is soft. Stir the chopped mushrooms and parsley into the cooked rice mixture. Stir in the lemon juice to season.

Chips in jackets: We all love chips, even though they are so full of fat and they are especially hard for children to give up. Instead of banning them altogether, try this low-fat recipe which is a much healthier alternative.

1 tbsp olive oil
1 tsp garlic purée or garlic oil
450g (1lb) large potatoes, scrubbed

Preheat the oven to 200°C (gas mark 6, 400°F). Mix together the olive oil and garlic. Use a sharp knife to slice the potatoes lengthways in half, then into long segments, like an orange. Place the potato 'chips' onto a non-stick baking tray. Brush with the oil and garlic mixture and lightly season with pepper. Bake in a preheated oven for 30–40 minutes, or until golden brown.

Healthy hash browns: This is a low-fat version of American's favourite fried potato dish. Always use organically grown potatoes when possible as they are not sprayed with antisprouting chemicals which do not wash off. Adults may prefer these with a touch of cayenne pepper added to the mixture before cooking.

2 tbsps olive oil
450g (1lb) potatoes, scrubbed
1 medium onion, finely chopped
2 cloves of garlic, crushed and chopped
1 tbsp chopped fresh parsley to garnish

Heat the oil in a large frying pan, wiping away any excess with kitchen paper towel. Add the onions and garlic and stir well. Cut the potatoes into thin slices and add to the oil. Press down with the back of a wooden spoon and sprinkle with pepper to taste. Cover the pan with a lid and turn down the heat so the potatoes gently cook through. Once cooked, turn the heat up to brown them on the outside. Divide the potatoes in half and flip

BABY AND TODDLER FOOD

over to brown the other side. Remove from the pan and blot on kitchen paper towel to remove all excess oil before serving.

Frozen pea fritters: These bright green fritters taste delicious and particularly appeal to children. They are full of fibre and vitamins and are also fun to make, so get the kids to help. Serve with grilled tomatoes or topped with a spoonful of passata (sieved tomatoes).

225g (8oz) frozen peas
1 egg, separated
1/4 tsp (a pinch of) cayenne pepper
100g (4oz) chick pea (gram) flour
pinch of salt

Preheat the oven to 160°C (gas mark 3, 325°F). Defrost the frozen peas by piercing a hole in the bag and cooking on medium in the microwave for 1–2 minutes. Alternatively, simmer the frozen peas in boiling water for 3–4 minutes. Remove from the heat and drain. Place the peas, egg yolk and cayenne pepper in a food processor and whizz until the mixture resembles a thick paste. Beat the egg white until stiff and stir into the mixture. Stir flour into mixture and shallow fry on both sides. Drain on kitchen paper and keep the first batch warm in the oven while you cook the rest.

FRUIT AND PUDDINGS

Fruit always makes an excellent dessert. Try the more exotic varieties or make a simple fruit salad from satsuma segments and chopped apple. The other quick, easy and ideal pudding is yoghurt. The best (and cheapest) way is to buy big tubs of natural yoghurt and flavour with some fruit juice, pieces of fresh or dried fruit, fruit purées or chopped nuts. The following recipes are all good ideas for puddings to add some variety every now and then.

RECIPES

Fruit salad: Any fruits can be used in a fruit salad, so the cheapest way of making this is to use whatever is in season at the time. Or for a special treat you could make an exotic fruit salad with all the tropical fruits. This is a good basic fruit salad – always leave edible skins on fruit as a valuble source of vitamins and fibre.

½ pint orange juice
2 oranges, peeled and cut into chunks
1 red apple, cored and cut into chunks
1 pear, cored and cut into chunks
1 small bunch seedless grapes, halved
1 kiwi fruit, peeled, halved lengthways and sliced
1 banana, sliced

Put the orange juice in a bowl and chop the fruit into it. Begin with the oranges as they will then stop the apple and pear turning brown. Add the banana just before serving as it goes brown after slicing.

Apricot and apple jelly: This is a wonderfully bright and fresh jelly. It is also slightly wobbly, so if you want to turn your jelly out from its mould use about ¾ pint of mixed juices. A vegetarian version may be made by using an agar gelling agent available from health-food shops.

300ml (½ pint) apple juice
300ml (½ pint) apricot juice
1 sachet or 3 tsps powdered gelatine
1 passion fruit, pulped (optional)

Mix the apple and apricot juices together. Put about one-third of the mixture into a bowl. Evenly sprinkle in the gelatine and gently heat over a pan of hot water until all the gelatine has dissolved. Slowly add the remaining fruit juice while stirring (do not add the gelatine mixture to the fruit juice). Cover and chill until set. Serve decorated with the pulped passion fruit (optional).

BABY AND TODDLER FOOD

Mandarin jelly: This jelly is a wonderfully nutritious and tasty alternative to the chunks of gelatine sold in supermarkets.

1 tin (300g) mandarins in juice
¾ pint orange juice
1 sachet or 3 tsps powdered gelatine

Drain the juice from the mandarins and mix with the orange juice. Place about half the liquid in a bowl and sprinkle in the gelatine. Heat gently until all the gelatine has dissolved. Add the remaining juice bit by bit, stirring continuously. Leave to cool for a couple of minutes, then sprinkle in the mandarins (they will sink down). Cover and chill until set.

Raspberry iced yoghurt: Raspberries are my favourites, but this recipe works with many fruits. All the berry fruits look and taste great, but for a more delicate flavour try peach or pear.

6 tbsps plain yoghurt (Greek-style is especially good)
12 tbsps raspberry purée (see page 55)
1 banana, mashed

Half freeze the yoghurt in a large plastic basin. Combine the banana and raspberry purée, then mix thoroughly into the semi-frozen yoghurt. Return to the freezer. In the next 1–1½ hours, take the yoghurt out a couple of times and beat with a fork to break up any ice crystals, and then return it to the freezer. Allow to soften for 10 minutes at room temperature before serving.

Strawberry sorbet: This recipe can be easily adapted for use with other soft fruits, such as raspberries. While it's great for children on a summer afternoon, it can also add the finishing touch to a smart supper.

450g (1lb) fresh strawberries
juice of 1 large orange

Blend the ingredients together in a food processor until smooth. Pour into a bowl or container and place in the freezer for 1

RECIPES

hour. Remove and allow the mixture to thaw slightly, if necessary, then beat well with a metal spoon to break up any ice crystals and return the sorbet to the freezer for at least 5 hours. Allow to soften at room temperature for half an hour before serving.

Apple crumble: Use eating apples for their natural sweetness. Serve the crumble with fromage frais or with iced yoghurt.

> 450g (1lb) eating apples, peeled, cored and sliced
> 1 tsp grated lemon rind
> 1/2 tsp cinnamon
> 25g (1oz) wholewheat, plain flour
> 25g (1oz) ground almonds
> 75 g (3oz) rolled oats
> 1 tbsp sesame seeds
> 4 tbsps sesame or olive oil

Preheat the oven to 160°C (gas mark 3, 325°F). Place the apples in a lightly oiled, shallow baking dish. Sprinkle with the lemon rind. Sift the flour, cinnamon and ground almonds into a basin and stir in the oats. Add the oil and mix with a wooden spoon until crumbly. Sprinkle the crumble topping over the apple and bake for 30 minutes or until the apples are tender.

Nice rice pudding: This wonderfully warming pudding gets most of its sweetness from the sweet brown rice. It is important to use precooked rice.

> 100g (4oz) cooked sweet brown rice
> 1 tbsp sultanas
> 600ml (1 pint) skimmed soya milk
> 1/2 tsp grated nutmeg (optional)

Preheat the oven to 150°C (gas mark 2, 300°F). Mix the precooked rice and sultanas and place in a lightly oiled ovenproof dish. Pour the soya milk evenly over the rice. Sprinkle the nutmeg on top. Bake for approximately 2 hours. *Note:* Nutmeg is a hallucinogenic spice and should not be given to babies.

BABY AND TODDLER FOOD

Prune brulée: This deliciously sweet pudding recipe looks and tastes like a cross between crème caramel and crème brulée but it is much lower in fat and sugar. It is especially popular with small children and the quantities given here will make a large dishful.

> 1/2 tsp sunflower oil
> 100g (4oz) brown sugar
> 300g (11oz) pitted prunes
> 2 eggs
> 1 tsp natural vanilla extract
> 40g (1 1/2 oz) wholewheat flour
> 250ml (8fl oz) skimmed milk
> 275ml (9fl oz) low-fat fromage frais

Preheat the oven to 190°C (gas mark 5, 375°F). Lightly oil a 23cm or 9" ceramic or glass pie dish. Sprinkle 2 tablespoons of the sugar inside the dish and tilt to coat the surfaces. Arrange the prunes on top. In a blender, combine the eggs, natural vanilla extract and remaining sugar. Blend until smooth. Add the flour and mix briefly. Add the milk and fromage frais and blend until smooth. Pour the mixture into the dish and bake for about 45 minutes until puffed and browned.

DRINKS

Wake-up shake: This wake-up shake will boost your child's vitamin levels and give kids extra energy at the start of the day. It tastes best chilled, so keep your milk or apple juice in the fridge before using. The blackstrap molasses give the shake a delicious tang and are also a useful source of iron.

> 1 level tbsp sunflower seeds
> 1 level tbsp sesame seeds
> 150ml (1/4 pint) skimmed milk or apple juice
> 1 tsp crude blackstrap molasses
> 1 ripe banana, peeled (optional)

Finely grind the seeds in a coffee mill (extra supplies may be ground and stored in the fridge to save preparation time). Blend the ground seeds, milk or apple juice, molasses and banana (if using) together in food mixer or liquidiser. Serve immediately while still frothy.

Mango and banana shake: This simple shake is a delicious way to top up on vitamins.
1 ripe banana, peeled
1 ripe mango, peeled and pitted (or portion of cantaloupe melon)
300ml (½ pint) skimmed milk

Mix all the ingredients together in a food processor or blender to create a deliciously frothy shake.

Strawberry and pineapple shake: This shake gets the taste-buds tingling and is a great idea for breakfast or elevenses. The strawberries are packed full of vitamin C, potassium and fibre.
150g (6fl oz) fresh strawberries
120g (4fl oz) pineapple juice
100g (4oz) plain low-fat, live yoghurt

Wash and hull the strawberries. Place in a blender or food processor. Pour on the pineapple juice and yoghurt. Whizz until smooth. Serve as a drink in a tall tumbler, or pour over muesli or granola-style cereal.

Sunny sundae: This is a great way to sneak some beta-carotene and extra vitamins into your child's diet. This drink is particularly good if you use freshly squeezed juices.
150ml (¼ pint) orange juice
150ml (¼ pint) carrot juice
Orange slice to decorate

Mix the two juices and chill. Decorate with orange slices before serving.

BABY AND TODDLER FOOD

Party Food

Sandwiches: The traditional mainstay of party teas, sandwiches are also nutritionally sound. Use your imagination with fillings, using a variety of lean meat, boneless fish, well-cooked eggs, fruit and vegetables. Don't forget the peanut butter! It is a good idea to bind the ingredients together with yoghurt or fromage frais (much lower in fat than mayonnaise or salad dressing). Wholemeal bread is best, but stripy sandwiches are fun with one side white and one brown. Sandwich shapes also go down a treat. Try cutting the sandwiches with novelty cutters and watch little hands grab their favourite animals.

Finger food: Fingers of fruit and vegetables are packed full of vitamins and wonderfully colourful. Carrots, broccoli, cauliflower, sweet pepper (assorted colours), celery, cucumber, apple, orange segments and seedless grapes. Mix in some strips of cheddar cheese as a contrasting taste and texture. Bread sticks and rice cakes are also good for nibbles. Popcorn is an eternal winner (see below) – and little children enjoy it just as much plain without any sugar or salt. Little pizza biscuits are another excellent idea – see Pizza-issimo on the next page.

Bowls of dried fruit are excellent for sweeter nibbles, especially dates, raisins and sultanas which are less tough to chew. Make the delicious fruity truffles (see below), although you may have trouble keeping the adults off them long enough for them to reach the party table.

Popcorn: Popcorn is also wonderful fun to make on a rainy afternoon and children of all ages love being in on the 'popping'. Heat 1 tablespoon of vegetable oil (olive oil is particularly good, being high in vitamin E and stable at high temperatures) in a large saucepan. Add 25g (1oz) of popping corn. Place the lid on the pan tightly and hold it on while shaking the pan. Only lift the lid once most of the popping has stopped. Serve warm or cold.

Pizza-issimo:

> 1 packet of oatcakes (read the label as some versions are very high in salt and fat)
> 4 tbsps passata (sieved tomatoes)
> 1 clove of garlic, crushed
> dash of Worcestershire sauce
> 75g (3oz) medium cheddar cheese, finely grated
> 1 tbsp fresh parsley, chopped

Mix the passata, garlic and Worcestershire sauce together. Spread over the oatcakes. Sprinkle the cheese and parsley over the top. Place under a hot grill for a couple of minutes, or until the cheese is completely melted and browning slightly at the edges.

Fruity truffles:

> 225g (8oz) dried fruit (apricots, dates, pears, raisins, etc)
> 25g (1oz) ground almonds
> 2 tbsps apple juice
> 50g (2oz) sesame seeds

Place the fruit, almonds and apple juice in a blender or food processor and work together until you have a smooth, quite stiff paste. Roll spoonfuls of the mixture into bite-sized balls and coat them in sesame seeds (the easiest way is to roll them in a small bowl of sesame seeds). Chill them in the fridge before freezing until hard. Serve cold.

Puddings: A good party tip is to opt for a healthy version of the traditional jelly and ice-cream. See the recipes for mandarin jelly and iced yoghurt (page 78).

BISCUITS AND CAKES

Birthday fruit cake: What party is complete without the all-important cake? Decorate this exceptionally moist cake with a ribbon round the outside and matching candles. Strips of marzipan work a treat for writing or a design on the top.

BABY AND TODDLER FOOD

275g (10oz) currants
275g (10oz) sultanas
350g (12oz) raisins
150g (5oz) chopped dried dates
100g (4oz) chopped dried apricots
450ml (³/₄ pint) orange juice
2 oranges, zest and juice
2 lemons, zest only
200g (7oz) butter
50g (2oz) brown sugar
4 eggs
1 tbsp malt extract
¹/₂ banana, mashed
100g (4oz) chopped mixed nuts
175g (6oz) wholemeal flour
50g (2oz) ground almonds
1 tsp dried ginger
1 tsp cinnamon
2 tsps mixed spice

Leave the dried fruit to soak in the orange juice with the lemon and orange zest for at least an hour. Cream the butter and sugar together. Beat in the eggs two at a time. Blend in the malt extract and banana. Stir in the chopped nuts, fruit and orange juice. Combine the remaining dry ingredients and fold in a bit at a time. Line a 25cm/10" round tin with greaseproof paper and grease. Bake in a preheated oven at 160°C (gas mark 3, 325°F) for about 2 hours or until a knife comes out clean. Cool on a wire rack.

Flapjacks: These taste absolutely delicious cut into fingers and dunked in various fruit purées, especially apple.

125ml (4fl oz) sunflower or walnut oil
2 tbsps clear honey
1 tbsp malt extract
2 tbsps date purée (see page 48)

125g (4oz) jumbo oats
125g (4oz) rolled oats
25g (1oz) sunflower seeds
25g (1oz) sesame seeds
40g (1½ oz) sultanas

Heat the oil, honey and malt extract gently, stirring until combined. Still stirring add the date purée and heat until evenly mixed. Remove from the heat and add the other ingredients, and mix thoroughly. Press into a greased (with some of the vegetable oil) 20 x 30cm baking tray. Bake in a preheated oven at 180°C (gas mark 4, 350°F) for half an hour. Take out and allow to cool slightly before cutting into squares. Leave in the baking tray to finish cooling.

Nutty cookies:
4 tbsps walnut oil (or sunflower oil)
2 tbsps clear honey
50g (2oz) peanut butter
1 egg
25g (1oz) rolled oats
50g (2oz) plain wholemeal flour
25g (1oz) ground almonds
1 tsp baking powder
25g (1oz) chopped nuts of your choice, browned
25g (1oz) sunflower seeds, browned

Stir the oil, honey and peanut butter together over a gentle heat until combined. Add all of the other ingredients and mix well. Place small spoonfuls of the mixture on a greased baking sheet, leaving space for them to spread. Bake in a preheated oven at 180°C (gas mark 4, 350°F) for 12–15 minutes. Leave to cool on a wire rack.

5
Special Diets

Many people eat a restricted diet either out of choice or because they suffer from some kind of allergy. It is important when following any diet which differs from the norm to ensure that you include all the important nutrients, vitamins and minerals. We should be especially aware of children's special needs and ensure that they receive their fair share of nutrients.

The Vegetarian Baby

Vegetarian food is delicious and even the most ardent carnivore benefits from eating vegetarian dishes as part of everyday food. A healthy balanced diet is easy to achieve for your baby and toddler provided you give it some thought and care. It is not enough to simply cut out all meat and fish, unless you replace all the valuable nutrients they contain.

Eating enough protein is particularly important for babies and young children as it is such an important nutrient for growth and development, especially of the brain. For a vegetarian child, the two major sources of complete protein, meat and fish, are eliminated from the diet. So eggs, dairy products and soya products should be eaten as these all contain complete protein. Soya beans have as much protein as top quality steak, but with the advantage of only containing unsaturated fats. Incomplete protein is also valuable, although greater quantities have to be consumed. This is because incomplete protein does not contain all the essential amino acids needed by the growing body. Different foods contain different amino acids. By provid-

SPECIAL DIETS

ing a wide variety of vegetarian foods you will guarantee your child gets his or her full quota. Incomplete protein is found in beans, peas, lentils, nuts, grains and cereals.

To make complete protein from incomplete proteins eat:

* Legumes with grains/nuts and seeds.
* Grains with legumes/dairy products.
* Nuts and seeds with legumes.

Iron intake is also important. Sufficient should be obtained easily from eating plenty of soya products and eggs. But it is worth choosing breakfast cereals fortified with iron. Certain cereals are also fortified with some of the B complex vitamins which may be very valuable, so check the packet. Vegetarians may be at risk of a vitamin B12 deficiency so you should consider a supplement. In a vegetarian diet zinc is not easily absorbed, so plenty of wheatgerm and green and yellow vegetables should be incorporated in the diet to remedy this.

The Vegan Baby

Strictly vegan diets are difficult to manage for a baby or toddler. They should only be undertaken if you have a thorough knowledge of nutrition. Vegans do not eat any animal products, so dairy products and eggs are eliminated from the diet in addition to meat and fish. This makes it very hard to obtain a good all-round nutritional intake. A balanced vegan diet is possible in theory, with nut and soya milks and synthetic supplements, but it is actually very difficult to obtain enough calcium, iron, riboflavin, vitamin B12 and vitamin D for healthy development. Children on vegan diets normally have a lower weight and, more worryingly, a lower than average height. If a child's bone structure has not reached its full potential size then the skull and brain might not have fully developed. All such highly restricted

BABY AND TODDLER FOOD

diets should be undertaken with great care and, in the case of young children, only with qualified guidance.

Diets for Allergies

An allergy occurs when there is an adverse reaction to something we eat, drink, inhale or touch. The most common symptoms are eczema, asthma and hayfever. Less usual are problems such as migraines, stomach upsets and catarrh. It is often difficult to pinpoint the offending article that triggers the problem. This is because allergies are also affected by our emotional state, tiredness, stress and general well-being, so symptoms can at some times be severe and at others very mild. To further confuse us, it is often quite common for one symptom to have several causes.

The most common food allergens for small children are cow's milk, cheese, eggs, fish, wheat, dried fruits, bananas, citrus fruits, nuts (especially almonds), chocolate and artificial food colouring and additives. These foods should be restricted in the diets of very young babies to try to prevent the development of an allergy.

ECZEMA AND ASTHMA

Eczema is a distressingly common skin condition. Signs of eczema are red and itchy skin with small blisters. As these heal the skin becomes tough and extremely dry. Asthma is a related disorder and occurs when the air passages in the lungs narrow during an attack, making breathing difficult, laboured and wheezing. It must be remembered that asthma is often a reaction to non-dietary factors such as passive smoking and pollution. However, the chief food culprits for both of these conditions tend to be cow's milk and eggs, possibly cheese, yoghurt, butter and cream. All should be eliminated from the diet. If you do remove these from your child's diet, it is advisable to give supplements to replace their calcium and vitamin D supplies. Replacements for cow's milk include goat's milk, soya milk and nut milks. For the dairy products, again use sheep or goat's milk products and any soya products. Vegetable oils and soya margarines can be used instead of butter. In fact, using some vegetable oil in the diet every day has in some cases been positively beneficial for eczema sufferers. Eggs are quite easy to avoid, as egg-less variations of many of the foods normally containing egg are simple to make. However, eggs do have a habit of hiding in readymade foods, so check the labels. As breast-fed babies have a lower incidence of eczema and asthma it is especially worthwhile breast feeding your baby if there is a history of these allergies in the family.

COELIAC DIET

This is where a person has an intolerance to gluten. The gluten irritates the small intestine lining and reduces its ability to absorb foods. Symptoms are persistent diarrhoea, stomach pain and a sharp drop in weight. Gluten is primarily found in wheat, but sufferers may also have to eliminate rye, barley and oats from the diet. This diet does not present a particular problem in nutritional terms, but can be fiddly as so many foods contain wheat or wheat flour. The only problem could be low levels of dietary fibre, so plenty of brown rice, pulses and vegetables must be eaten. Increasing numbers of alternatives to wheat and flour are becoming available. These include maize, millet, rice and buckwheat. For readymade dishes, keep your eyes open for the gluten-free symbol of a crossed grain. It is worth getting in touch with the Coeliac Society who produce an annually updated list of gluten-free manufactured foods (see *Useful Addresses*). Gluten-free flour can also be bought from some chemists and health-food shops. Ground rice, chick pea flour and corn flour can also be used.

BABY AND TODDLER FOOD

HYPERACTIVITY – THE FEINGOLD DIET

This diet was formulated by the late Dr Ben Feingold, an American allergist. He spent many years researching the possible link between chemical food additives, hyperactivity and behavioural disturbances. Dr Feingold believed that changes in the diet are preferable to drugs as a method for helping children with such problems, as drugs only eliminate the symptom and not the cause. Symptoms of hyperactivity include continuous motion (eg rocking and leg wriggling), needing very little sleep, self-abusiveness and aggression, excessive tantrums, erratic and disruptive behaviour, clumsy movements, feeding problems and poor appetite. Hyperactive children may also resist cuddling and affection, and have a complete lack of concentration.

Two groups of foods should be eliminated from the diet.

Group One: All fruit and vegetables which contain high levels of natural salicylates: *Almonds, apples, apricots, berries, cherries, cucumbers, currants, grapes and raisins, green peppers, nectarines, oranges (Note: grapefruits, lemons and limes are allowed), peaches, plums and prunes, tomatoes.* These fruits and vegetables must be completely omitted, including any foodstuffs which contain any of these as an ingredient.

Group Two: Any foods containing artificial colourings and flavourings. The coal-tar dyes such as tartrazine (E102) and sunset yellow (E110) are especially common allergens. BHT (butylated hydroxytoluene) must also be omitted. This means careful reading of any labels on shop-bought food. Many foods may have to be prepared at home from fresh ingredients to avoid these common additives.

6
Commercial Foods

Preschool children consume well over 50 million meals each week. This enormous eating capacity greatly interests the food giants and it is small wonder that children have become such a target for manufacturers. Sales of baby food and drink alone account for more than £150 million a year, which works out at an average of more than £200 per baby per year. The toddler food market is even more lucrative at £250 million a year. The market has been well targeted. In the government's *Dietary Survey of Infants Aged Six to Twelve Months*, it was found that 82 percent of British babies consumed some commercial food (excluding formula milks), which means that only 18 percent rely on 'home-prepared' foods alone.

The Baby Drinks Horror Story

Most dentists are familiar with rampant tooth decay in babies. This is now such a common phenomenon that it has been given its own name – 'nursing bottle caries'. This is a painful, disfiguring condition which in extreme cases reduces babies' soft teeth to blackened stumps. The damage can have a knock-on effect far into the future and a child's second set of teeth can be permanently malformed. There is also the possibility of speech problems and psychological problems stemming from toothlessness. If this sounds like scaremongering, bear in mind that in a single year 23,000 children aged four years' and under receive a general anaesthetic for multiple tooth extractions. Remember that this figure is indicative of the volume of

BABY AND TODDLER FOOD

only the more serious cases, so the problem is therefore very widespread.

This huge problem has one main cause: sugared drinks. Nursing bottle caries are caused by prolonged, frequent or late-night consumption of sugared drinks in a baby bottle or training cup, or dummies dipped in honey or concentrated fruit juices. These drinks are specifically marketed for babies and young children, or sold as 'healthy' drinks or cordials. However, the link between these drinks and infant tooth decay is so strong that more than 600 families are suing the five major UK manufacturers over injuries to their children's teeth. A central issue in this legal action is the inadequacy of labelling leading to risks of misuse. So, just because a product has a picture of a baby with a toothy grin on the label, do not assume that it will make your baby happy in the long run.

Fortunately consumer pressure together with the threat of legal action, a potential boycott and a future EC directive have forced some changes in the products available. Manufacturers have started to reduce the amount of sugar in such products and some have even put warnings on the packets. However, low sugar is not good enough, as it still contains *some form* of sugar. Dentists have pointed out that it is not the total amount of sugar, but the length of time that the teeth are exposed to sugar which is the relevant factor in tooth decay. This point is worth remembering for any other sugar eaten and dentists encourage eating sweet things all at one time instead of snacking throughout the day. It was heartening to see the recent introduction of the first sugar-free varieties of baby drinks, with Boots and Milupa leading the way. However, make sure that your baby's drinks do not contain artificial sweeteners either, such as saccharin and aspartame. Many medics believe that adding a daily dose of such chemicals to our diet is potentially dangerous and some of the artificial sweeteners are known to be carcinogenic (cancer-causing) in large quantities.

COMMERCIAL FOODS

The Health Education Authority's advice on drinks for your baby is clear. Under six months' old, nothing other than breast or formula milk and cooled, boiled water (only where necessary) should be given. Once a baby is over six months' old, he or she can also be given very diluted fruit juice. The HEA does not recommend any other drinks for babies; however, it does add that no sweetened drink should ever be left with children in bottles or reservoir feeders.

Nutritious Baby Food?

Processed baby foods come in two forms – packets of dry powder to which you just add milk or water and jars of ready-to-eat blended food. Unfortunately, the contents of many packets and jars are not necessarily as wholesome as they first appear. All processed food loses some nutritional value in its manufacture and often the food bulk is provided by highly refined starches and sugars which provide 'empty calories'. Many packet foods contain vitamins that have been synthetically manufactured which may not be as well absorbed and utilised by the body as the nutrients that occur naturally in food. Jars of ready-to-eat food tend to offer a better deal. It is interesting to note that a common ingredient at the top of the label list (and therefore the greatest ingredient) is water. This is then combined with a thickening agent which appears further down the list, as only small amounts are needed. It is almost impossible to gauge what percentage of these products is simply thickened water. Part of the problem is that manufacturers are not obliged to put the proportions of different ingredients on the label. There is little comparison between what is readily available in packets and jars and the fresh food you can make for your baby yourself.

Fortunately, a few companies are beginning to make improvements. This is very welcome as there is no doubt that

BABY AND TODDLER FOOD

convenience foods can be useful additions to the store cupboard. The health-food shop is often the best place to look for healthier options. Supermarkets are slowly getting better too and some even stock organic baby food ranges which tend to have a better list of ingredients and are made without cheap bulking agents and starchy fillers.

Reading the Labels

Knowledge is power. If you know what is in a food, you can choose whether or not you want your family to eat it. Knowledge gives you control over the nutritional health of your nearest and dearest. Therefore, I urge you to begin this one simple lifelong habit when buying any food and that is to READ THE LABELS before you buy. Although food labels can initially be a maze of unknown words and chemical names, it soon becomes easy to negotiate your way around the jargon to the end goal of a nutritious meal.

QUICK TIPS

* Ignore the flashy messages on the front of a packet – these can often be misleading. Those that boldly claim 'low in fat' may not be so forthright about being 'high in sugar'.
* Turn the item over and read the actual ingredients. These are listed in order of amount, so if one of the nutrition nasties is high up the list, maybe this food isn't such a good idea.
* An easy way of selecting a brand is to rule out those foods with a long list of chemical names. The foods with the most ingredients which can be recognised as actual foods are likely to be the closest to a home-made recipe and are probably more wholesome.

COMMERCIAL FOODS

SUGAR SHOCKS
Manufacturers have become very devious about making the amount of sugar added to a product appear a lot less than it really is. This is especially worrying when we are trying not to develop potential sweet tooths in tiny mouths. Surprisingly, sugar is added to a huge number of foods, including many savory foods where you might not expect to find it. There are also many common foods which always contain sugar, for example, until recently it was impossible to buy baked beans without added sugar. With other common foods that is still often the case.

SUGARY TACTICS
* In the ingredients list, sugar is often split up into more than one type so it appears several times further down the list. This may fool you into believing there is less total sugar. Look for any of the substances mentioned below, but the quick guide is to keep your eyes peeled for any names which include sucrose, glucose, dextrose or syrup.
* Sugar has many guises – sucrose, glucose, dextrose, glucose syrup, dried glucose syrup, corn syrup, hydrogenated glucose syrup, fructose, lactose, honey, invert syrup, maple syrup, golden syrup, molasses and dark treacle. All of these are empty calories and could develop a sweet tooth.
* 'Low sugar' – but the very fact that it says low sugar means it contains some sugar. It is only in relation to another similar, but high sugar, product that it has any meaning. So beware – babies' rusks which have been sold as low sugar products may have more sugar than your average doughnut!
* 'No added sugar' – this could mean a sweetener by another name has been added, eg concentrated fruit juice or lactose.

BABY AND TODDLER FOOD

* 'No artificial sweeteners' – this may well mean that natural sweeteners, ie sugars, have been added. However, it is useful to know that artificial sweeteners are banned from baby foods, so while it is fine to put this message on their packaging, the manufacturers are only stating that they have done what they are obliged to do by law! Remember that many foods or drinks you give to your youngsters are not necessarily marketed for babies or young children and may therefore contain artificial sweeteners, such as aspartame (Nutrasweet), saccharin, sorbitol (E420), mannitol (E421), xylitol and hydrogenated glucose syrup, so watch out for these.

COLOURINGS AND PRESERVATIVES

'No artificial colourings' – this may well imply that natural colourings have been added. What counts as natural in a food may surprise you. In the case of colourings, cochineal is deemed natural, but did you know that it comes from the eggs and ovaries of the cactus beetle? By law, no artificial or natural colourings should be added to baby and toddler foods apart from three which are also vitamins. These are riboflavin (E101), riboflavin-5'-phosphate (E101a), and carotene (E160a), all various orange-yellow colours. Sometimes other foods, such as caramel, grape skins and blackcurrants, are added as colouring. This is a very valid part of cooking and cooks throughout the ages have added coloured foodstuffs for interest and variety. Bear in mind though, that the more added colour (and taste and texture) in a food, the less wholesome and more refined it is likely to be.

All foods which are intended to be kept for a time need either a preservative or some type of treatment to prevent them from going off. We come across many of these every day, for instance pasteurisation, sterilisation, dehydration, vacuum packing and freezing. Preservatives which are added are listed as 'E numbers' (see *Additive Decoder* overleaf). In addition, ascorbic acid (vitamin C), salt, vinegar and concentrated sugar may also be added as preservatives but do not come under this heading on the label. If food is to be kept safely it does need preserving, but fresh is nutritionally best, so where possible use fresh foods. Some preservatives are banned from baby foods and these include nitrates and nitrites which are normally found in cured meats and sausages (so read the label before you give these to your toddler).

WHAT IS NATURAL?

Many packets, bottles and jars on the supermarket shelves bear the inscription 'only natural ingredients'. But many things are natural and this doesn't necessarily mean they are good to eat. While carrots, chicken and apples are all natural, so are salt, sugar, even wood and arsenic! In fact, the word 'natural' covers ingredients found in insects, crab shells, bird feathers, cotton and wood. Even foodstuffs synthetically manufactured in a laboratory can be called natural, or 'nature identical' if they are found in a similar form in nature. So the word 'natural' on a label does not necessarily mean 'wholesome'.

THE E NUMBERS

Everything consists entirely of chemicals including all the food we eat. However, as we well know, there are a whole bunch of chemicals which manufacturers add to processed foods as 'additives'. Some of these are genuinely necessary for the roles of preserving foods and protecting them from contamination, but the vast majority are added to the food for cosmetic reasons. In fact, 88 percent of the additive budget is spent on these colourings, flavourings, flavour enhancers and sweeteners. A further 11 percent is spent on chemicals whose sole role is to make the recipe or processing method work effectively, such as thickeners. This leaves a pathetic 1 percent used for the valid role of food preservation.

BABY AND TODDLER FOOD

Many additives have been allocated an infamous E number. This simply means that they have been approved for use throughout the European Community. But while they have been officially approved as safe, there may be reasons why certain additives are unsuitable for some groups of people. Just as some natural foods, such as strawberries or peanuts, can cause an allergic reaction or adverse effect, so might some of these chemicals. Below are listed the possible culprits which can cause problems or worsen allergic conditions. Those with asthma, hyperactivity, aspirin sensitivity and phenylketonuria (PKU) should all take especial care. Although many are banned from baby and toddler foods (such as all the colourings) it is still worth keeping your eyes peeled and remember that fewer additives are banned from 'grown-up' foods which could well be offered to a small child. Manufacturers have grown wise to the fact that many of us are suspicious of E numbers and may list the additives under their name – so beware if there is a string of long chemical names in the ingredients list. As a rule of thumb, I do not buy anything with an ingredient name that I do not understand or cannot pronounce!

The following table lists additives you should watch out for and the reasons why.

Table 10
Additive decoder

COLOURINGS

E102 Tartrazine – one of the most common colourings to trigger adverse reactions, such as hyperactivity and eczema.

E104 Quinoline yellow – may provoke similar adverse reactions in sensitive people.

COMMERCIAL FOODS

E110 Sunset yellow FCF (orange yellow S) – may provoke similar adverse reactions in sensitive people.

E120 Cochineal (carminic acid) – may provoke allergic reactions.

E122 Carmoisine (azorubine) – may provoke adverse reactions in sensitive people.

E123 Amaranth (red 2) – may provoke adverse reactions in sensitive people.

E124 Ponceau 4R (cochineal red R) – may provoke adverse reactions in sensitive people.

E127 Erythrosine – may provoke adverse reactions in sensitive people. In tests it has damaged thyroid glands of laboratory rats. Only permitted in cocktails and candied cherries.

E128 Red 2g – possible hazard for people deficient in the red blood cell enzyme glucose-6-phosphate dehydrogenase.

E129 Allura red AC – may provoke adverse reactions in sensitive people.

E131 Patent blue V (acid blue 3) – may provoke adverse reactions in sensitive people.

E132 Indigo carmine (indigotine) – may provoke adverse reactions in sensitive people.

E133 Brilliant blue FCF – may provoke adverse reactions in sensitive people.

E142 Green S (lissamine green) – may provoke adverse reactions in sensitive people.

E150(c) Ammonia caramel – possible hazard to those deficient in vitamin B6 and with deficient white blood cells.

E151 Black PN (brilliant black BN, food black) – may provoke adverse reactions in sensitive people.

BABY AND TODDLER FOOD

E153 Carbon black (vegetable carbon) – some from mineral sources may contain small quanities of unpleasant organic compounds, including benzpyrenes and polynuclear aromatic hydrocarbons, known to cause cancer in laboratory animals.

E154 Brown FK (brown for kippers) – may provoke adverse reactions in sensitive people. Only permitted in smoked and cured fish such as kippers.

E155 Brown HT (chocolate brown HT) – may provoke adverse reactions in sensitive people.

E160(b) Annatto (annatto extracts, bixin, norbixin) – may provoke intolerance symptoms.

E161(g) Canthaxanthin – use in artificial-suntan pills was banned after it appeared to cause damage to the eyes of some users. May be present in some fish and poultry feed but doesn't appear on labels of resulting food.

E173 Aluminium (and aluminium compounds E520, E521, E522, E523, E541, E554, E556, E558, E559 and E573) – may be linked to Alzheimer's disease, a form of senile dementia. Only permitted in the external coating of confectionery and a few liqueurs.

E180 Pigment rubine (lithol rubine BK) – may provoke adverse reactions in sensitive people. Only permitted on the surface of cheese (remove rind before serving to children).

Preservatives

E210 Benzoic acid – may provoke allergic reactions.

E211 Sodium benzoate (benzoate of soda) – may provoke allergic reactions.

E212 Potassium benzoate – may provoke allergic reactions.

COMMERCIAL FOODS

E213 Calcium benzoate (monocalcium benzoate) – may provoke allergic reactions.

E214 Ethyl 4-hydroxybenzoate (ehtyl pára-hydroxybenzoate) – may provoke allergic reactions.

E215 Ethyl 4-hydroxybenzoate, sodium salt (sodium ethyl para-hydroxybenzoate) – may provoke allergic reactions.

E216 Propyl 4-hydroxybenzoate (propylparaben) – may provoke allergic reactions.

E217 Propyl 4-hydroxybenzoate, sodium salt (sodium propyl para-hydroxybenzoate) – may provoke allergic reactions.

E218 Methyl 4-hydroxybenzoate (methyl para-hydroxybenzoate, methylparaben) – may provoke allergic reactions.

E219 Methyl 4-hydroxybenzoate, sodium salt (sodium methyl para-hydroxybenzoate) – may provoke allergic reactions.

E220 Sulphur dioxide – may provoke adverse reactions in sensitive people, including those with asthma. Destroys vitamin B1 so is unsuitable for those who are poorly nourished.

E221 Sodium sulphite – may provoke adverse reactions in sensitive people, including those with asthma. Destroys vitamin B1 so is unsuitable for those who are poorly nourished.

E222 Sodium hydrogen sulphite (sodium bisulphite) – may provoke adverse reactions in sensitive people, including those with asthma. Destroys vitamin B1 so is unsuitable for those who are poorly nourished.

E223 Sodium metabisulphite – may provoke adverse reactions in sensitive people, including those with

BABY AND TODDLER FOOD

asthma. Destroys vitamin B1 so is unsuitable for those who are poorly nourished.

E224 Potassium metabisulphite – may provoke adverse reactions in sensitive people, including those with asthma. Destroys vitamin B1 so is unsuitable for those who are poorly nourished.

E226 Calcium sulphite – may provoke adverse reactions in sensitive people, including those with asthma. Destroys vitamin B1 so is unsuitable for those who are poorly nourished.

E227 Calcium bisulphite (calcium hydrogen sulphite) – may provoke adverse reactions in sensitive people, including those with asthma. Destroys vitamin B1 so is unsuitable for those who are poorly nourished.

E228 Potassium hydrogen sulphite (potassium bisulphite) – may provoke adverse reactions in sensitive people, including those with asthma. Destroys vitamin B1 so is unsuitable for those who are poorly nourished.

E230 Diphenyl (biphenyl, phenyl benzene) – may provoke adverse reactions in sensitive people. Only permitted on citrus fruit skins.

E231 Orthophenylphenol may provoke adverse reactions in sensitive people. Only permitted on citrus fruit skins.

E232 Sodium orthophenylphenate (sodium orthophenylphenol) – may provoke adverse reactions in sensitive people. Only permitted on citrus fruit skins.

E233 Thiabendazole (2-[thiazol-4-yl] benzimidazole) – subject of debate. Only permitted on apple skins, with limits on the levels of residues.

E235 Natamycin (pimaricin) – may provoke adverse reactions in sensitive people. Only permitted on some cheese rinds and salami-type sausage casings.

COMMERCIAL FOODS

E239 Hexamine (HMT, hexamethylene tetramine, methenamine) – in tests it increased tumour rates and produced reproductive problems in laboratory rats. Only permitted in provolone cheese.

E249 Potassium nitrite – should not be used in food for infants.

E250 Sodium nitrite – directly hazardous to young babies. Can combine with protein to form nitrosamines, which have caused cancer in laboratory rats.

E251 Sodium nitrate (saltpetre, nitre) – directly hazardous to young babies.

E252 Potassium nitrate – directly hazardous to young babies.

E261 Potassium acetate – possibly hazardous for those with damaged or failing kidneys.

E270 Lactic acid (D-lactic acid, L-lactic acid, DL-lactic acid) – only L-lactic acid should be used in foods for infants.

E280 Propionic acid (propanoic acid) – in tests caused pre-cancerous damage in the digestive tracts of some laboratory rats.

E281 Sodium propionate (sodium propanoate) – in tests caused pre-cancerous damage in the digestive tracts of some laboratory rats.

E282 Calcium propionate (calcium propanoate) – in tests caused pre-cancerous damage in the digestive tracts of some laboratory rats.

E283 Potassium propionate – in tests caused pre-cancerous damage in the digestive tracts of some laboratory rats.

E296 DL-malic acid and L-malic acid (apple acid) – DL-malic acid may be unsuitable for infants.

BABY AND TODDLER FOOD

Antioxidants

E310 Propyl gallate (propyl ester of gallic acid) – may provoke adverse reactions in sensitive people.

E311 Octyl gallate – may provoke adverse reactions in sensitive people.

E312 Dodecyl gallate – may provoke adverse reactions in sensitive people.

E320 Butylated hydroxyanisole (BHA) – may trigger hyperactivity in sensitive people. In tests has caused cancers in the forestomachs of laboratory rats.

E321 Butylated hydroxytoluene (BHT) – inconsistent test results concerning changes in the incidence of cancer.

Emulsifiers, stabilisers, thickeners

E336(i) Monopotassium tartrate – may be unsuitable for those with weak kidneys or liver.

E336(ii) Dipotassium tartrate – may be unsuitable for those with weak kidneys or liver.

E385 Calcium disodium ethylene diamine tetra-acetate (calcium disodium EDTA) – should not be used in foods for infants.

E405 Propane-1,2-diol alginate (propylene glycol alginate) – may provoke adverse reactions in sensitive people.

E406 Agar (agar-agar, Japanese isinglass) – may provoke adverse reactions in sensitive people.

E407 Carrageenan (Irish moss, furcellaran) – in tests caused digestive tract ulcers and reproduction problems in some laboratory animals.

E413 Tragacanth gum – may provoke severe allergic reactions.

E414 Gum arabic (gum acacia) – may provoke adverse reactions in sensitive people.

COMMERCIAL FOODS

E420(i) Sorbitol – acts as a laxative, so should not be used in foods for infants.

E420(ii) Sorbitol syrup – acts as a laxative, so should not be used in foods for infants.

E421 Mannitol (manna sugar, mannite) – acts as a laxative, so should not be used in foods for infants. Only permitted in baby foods when used as a carrier for other ingredients.

E431 Polyoxyethylene (40) monostearate – too few tests conducted. Only permitted in wine.

FLAVOUR ENHANCERS AND SWEETENERS

E626 Guanylic acid – may be unsuitable for those suffering from gout.

E627 Sodium guanylate (guanosine 5-[disodium phosphate]) – may be unsuitable for those with gout.

E628 Dipotassium guanylate – may be unsuitable for those suffering from gout.

E629 Calcium guanylate – may be unsuitable for those suffering from gout.

E630 Inosinic acid – may be unsuitable for those suffering from gout.

E631 Sodium 5'-inosinate – may be unsuitable for those suffering from gout.

E632 Dipotassium inosinate – may be unsuitable for those suffering from gout.

E633 Calcium inosinate – may be unsuitable for those suffering from gout.

E634 Calcium 5'-ribonucleotides – may be unsuitable for those suffering from gout.

E635 Sodium 5'-ribonucleotides – may be unsuitable for those suffering from gout.

BABY AND TODDLER FOOD

E636   Maltol – causes bacteria to mutate. Only permitted in chewing gum.

E950   Acesulfame-K – caused increased incidence of cancer in laboratory animals. Limits on the levels permitted.

E951   Aspartame – subject of debate.

E952   Cyclamates – previously banned in the UK.

E953   Isomalt – acts as a laxative, so should not be used in foods for infants.

E954   Saccharin – increases incidence of bladder cancer in some laboratory rats. Should not be used in foods for infants. Children and pregnant women should limit their intake.

E965(i)   Maltitol – acts as a laxative, so should not be used in foods for infants.

E965(ii)   Maltitol syrup – acts as a laxative, so should not be used in foods for infants.

E966   Lactitol – acts as a laxative, so should not be used in foods for infants.

E967   Xylitol – acts as a laxative, so should not be used in foods for infants.

OTHERS

E925   Chlorine – destroys vitamin E and should be avoided by the poorly nourished.

E926   Chlorine dioxide (chlorine peroxide) – destroys vitamin E and should be avoided by the poorly nourished.

E928   Benzoyl peroxide – may provoke adverse reactions in sensitive people.

E999   Quillaia extracts – may provoke gastrointestinal irritation.

E1200   Polydextrose – large doses have a marked laxative effect.

E1201   Polyvinyl pyrrolidone – subject to debate.

COMMERCIAL FOODS

Note: The above guidelines are subject to an EC review and may change or not come into effect until 1995.

Not all bad news

Although commercially bought baby and toddler foods are not generally as wholesome or nutritious as home-cooked foods, they are not all bad news. They do offer the very real benefit of convenience and are a boon when travelling without access to a fridge or boiling water. What could be easier than opening a small sterile pot of baby food. And while tinned spaghetti or baked beans may contain some sugar (though it is getting easier to buy them without), they are essentially good basic food. Some processed foods, such as frozen vegetables, are even downright healthy! Provided your toddler is not on a permanent high sugar or high fat diet, small amounts of either will do no harm.

You would need the patience of a saint and limitless preparation time to make your child's food freshly every single day. There is no question that commercial foods are extremely useful time savers. Here is a list of the foods and drinks that I keep to hand for my own baby and toddler.

The healthy store-cupboard:
* Packets of plain baby rice
* Packets of no-sugar baby muesli
* Weetabix and no-sugar Ready-Brek
* Rice cakes (no salt)
* Frozen vegetarian sausages
* Frozen sesame nuggets
* Tinned precooked brown rice
* Jars of plain fruit and vegetable purées
* Fizzy mineral water, low salt varieties such as Spa, Malvern and Highland Spring

BABY AND TODDLER FOOD

- Carrot, grape and apple juice
- Low-salt yeast extract spreads, such as Natex
- Frozen vegetables such as peas, broccoli, cauliflower and sprouts. These can often contain *more* vitamin C than fresh vegetables as they are frozen within an hour of picking
- Tinned tomatoes and other vegetables (don't forget to drain off the salty and sugary water)
- Baked beans and wholemeal pasta hoops
- Tinned fish such as tuna, salmon and sardines (look for the varieties tinned in water or a vegetable oil)
- Frozen fish and fish fingers
- Pasta (try the red and green varieties which contain tomato and spinach, and wholewheat or egg pastas)
- Pizzas or plain pizza bases to pile with home-made toppings.

There is also hope that the many healthy messages in the media are beginning to reach the manufacturers. Many moves towards healthier alternatives are already being seen. However, this is only a start and we still have a long way to go before some of the processed food on the shop shelves makes up the best daily diet for our children. But consumer pressure really does work and you can help by boycotting products you dislike or by writing letters to manufacturers, supermarkets, your local MP and even newspapers and magazines.

A good point to remember about any commercial foods is that none of them will do immediate or specific damage to your child. This does not mean you should feed your child on all these products all the time, but that an occasional lapse is not a problem. The biscuit tin tucked at the back of the cupboard can be a sanity saver when your kids are screaming – they want food and they want it now!

Useful Addresses

Action Against Allergy
24-26 High Street
Hampton Hill
Middlesex TW12 1PD

Action and Information on
Sugars
PO Box 190
Walton-on-Thames
Surrey KT12 2YN

Ameda
Unit 2, Belvedere Trading Est.
Taunton TA1 1BH
Telephone: 0823 336 362

Association of Breast-feeding
Mothers
26 Holmshaw Close
London SE26 4TH
Telephone: 081 778 4769

Baby Milk Action
23 St Andrew's Street
Cambridge CB2 3AX
Telephone: 0223 464420

British Dietetic Association
7th Floor, Elizabeth House
22 Suffolk Street, Queensway
Birmingham B1 1LS
Telephone: 021 643 5483

British Nutrition Foundation
15 Belgrave Square
London SW1 1JJ
Telephone: 071 235 4904

The Coeliac Society
PO Box 220
High Wycombe
Buckinghamshire HP11 2HY

Consumers' Association
2 Marylebone Road
London NW1 4DF
Telephone: 071 486 5544

The Food Commission
3rd Floor
5-11 Worship St
London EC2A 2BH
Telephone: 071 628 7774

Health Education Authority
Hamilton House
Mabledon Place
London WC1H 9TX
Telephone: 071 383 3833

Healthy Visitors' Association
50 Southwark Street
London SE1 1UN
Telephone: 071 378 7255

BABY AND TODDLER FOOD

Hyperactive Children's
Support Group
71 Whyke Lane
Chichester
West Sussex PO19 2LD
Telephone: 0903 725182

Infant and Dietetic Foods
Association/Food and Drink
Association
6 Catherine Street
London WC2B 5JJ
Telephone: 071 836 2460

La Leche League
27 Old Gloucester Street
London WC1N 3AP
Telephone: 071 242 1278

Maternity Alliance
15 Britannia Street
London WC1X 9JP
Telephone: 071 837 1265

National Childbirth Trust
Alexandra House
Oldham Terrace
Acton
London W3 6NH
Telephone: 081 992 8637

National Eczema Society
4 Tavistock Place
London WC1H 9RA
Telephone: 071 388 4097

Parents for Safe Food
3rd Floor
5-11 Worship Street
London EC2A 2BH
Telephone: 071 628 2442

Vegetarian Society of the
United Kingdom
Parkdale
Dunham Road
Altrincham
Cheshire WA14 4QG
Telephone: 061 928 0793

Index

Allergies, diets for 88-90

Babies, newborn 23–28
Babies, 4–6 months 28–32, 46–9
Babies, 6–9 months 32–5
    recipes for 49–56
Babies, 9–12 months 35–9
    recipes for 56–63
Babies, 12 months and up
    see Toddlers
Breast feeding 21, 23–7

Commercial foods 91–108

Diet and development 7–8
Diet and health 6–8

Milk, breast 23–7
Milk, formula 27–8

Nutrition 9–22
    harmful substances 20–2, 91–106
    macronutrients 10–14
    micronutrients 15–18
    nutritional requirements 22
    water 18–20

Toddlers, 12 months and up 39–41
    recipes for 63–85

Vegan baby 87
Vegetarian baby 86–7

Weaning 28–32, 42–3

RECIPES

Apple crumble 79
Apricot and apple jelly 77
Apricot and orange muesli 63

Baked Beans 59–60
Barley and vegetable soup 50
Bean and flour patties 69
Beautiful bangers 65
Beef and mushroom casserole 65–6
Bircher muesli 63
Birthday fruit cake 83–4
Biscuits and cakes 83–5

Carrot soup 74
Cauliflower cheese 72–3
Cereals 46, 49–50, 63–5
Chicken and broccoli bake 66
Chicken and courgette shells 61
Chicken and leek with baked potato 56
Chicken and mango salad 66–7
Chicken and orange with rice 57
Chicken casserole 51
Chicken purée 50
Chicken stock 51
Chicken with lentils and apple 52
Chips in jackets 75
Cod in tomato 53
Cod with apple 58
Cod with rice and spinach 53
Crumbed plaice 58–9

Drinks 80–1

BABY AND TODDLER FOOD

Fast fish risotto 68–9
Fish 52–3, 57–60, 67–9
Fish cakes 68
Fishy soup 67–8
Flapjacks 84–5
Frozen pea fritters 76
Fruit and puddings 47–9, 55–6, 63, 76–80, 83
Fruit salad 77
Fruity truffles 83

Granny's fish pie 57–8

Hummus 59

Liver, leek and potato 53

Mandarin jelly 78
Marvellous mince 56–7
Meat 50–3, 56–7, 61, 65–7

Nice rice pudding 79
Nut butter 69–70
Nutty cookies 85

Oat and vegetable medley 50

Party food 82–3
Pasta 60–1, 71–2
Pasta parcels 72
Pasta pomodoro 71
Pinto bean casserole 60
Pizza–issimo 83
Plaice with cauliflower and mushroom 53
Popeye pie 71–2
Prune brulée 80
Pulses and nuts 54, 59–60, 69–70
Puréed carrots with basil 61–2

Raspberry iced yogurt 78
Red pepper rafts 73–4

Soya bean bake 70
'Spag bol' 72
Strawberry sorbet 78
Sweet potato and mushroom risotto 74–5

Tomato and vegetable soup 62
Tuna and sweetcorn 60–1

Vegetables 47–9, 55, 61–2, 72–6

Watercress and spinach rice 62